essential stretch

essential stretch

a better way to flow through life

Michelle LeMay

A Perigee Book

ℙ

A Perigee Book
Published by The Berkley Publishing Group
A division of Penguin Group (USA) Inc.
375 Hudson Street
New York, New York 10014

Copyright © 2003 by Michelle LeMay
Text design by Richard Oriolo
Interior photos by Curtis McElhinney
Cover design by Liz Sheehan

FIRST EDITION: August 2003

LIBRARY OF CONGRESS CATALOGING-IN-PUBLICATION DATA

LeMay, Michelle.
    Essential stretch / Michelle LeMay.
        p.   cm.
    Includes index.
    ISBN 0-399-52893-8 (pbk.)
        1. Stretching exercises.   2. Physical fitness.
    3. Exercise.   I. Title.

RA781.63.L46   2003
613.7'1—dc21

                                        2002035516

PRINTED IN THE UNITED STATES OF AMERICA

10   9   8   7   6   5   4   3   2   1

contents

acknowledgments

First I would like to thank all of my students, for I have been encouraged and fed by your results. Your rewards have inspired me to continue developing this technique. I know I am blessed to have students so open and receptive. And I truly appreciate those of you who have shared your personal experiences with me.

To Mom and Dad, thanks for raising me with integrity and for not taking life too seriously. You've taught me the importance of relaxing and enjoying life.

Thanks to Nealie for always being there with your beautiful, lighthearted, playful energy and with open ears and a creative mind.

Muchas gracias, Alana, for rescuing my graphics on the proposal for this book and for your love and creativity.

Thank you, Arnel, for all your love and support and invaluable nutritional guidance. You've changed my life forever.

To Richard, thank you for being a major catalyst to my personal growth and for your undying love and support.

To my agent, Carol Mann, thank you for all of your support and for always being available to me.

To Sheila Curry Oakes, thank you for all of your expertise, for this wonderful opportunity, and for believing in this book.

To Terri Hennessy—you are an angel. Thank you so much for all of your hard work and great edits.

Thanks to Heidi Dvorak for your advice on organizing this book and your added spice.

Thank you, Dr. Tim, for always sharing your vast knowledge with me.

To Curtis, my photographer, I appreciate your mellow energy. Whether we are meditating or working, you are wonderful company.

Gokula, thanks for coming through for me. Your help in editing is much appreciated.

foreword

by Cory Everson

I met Michelle twelve years ago and the very day I met her she became my soul mate and best friend for life. There was an energy and magnetism about her very being that transcends any aura I have ever encountered. Since then we have worked together on over two hundred and fifty television shows, five mind/body fitness retreats, and ten videos. She has an uncanny ability to read a person's energy and needs and creates a beautifully inviting atmosphere for self-expression, personal growth, and self-awareness. One's health goes much deeper than body fat or the fitness parameters of traditional testing techniques. Her stretch technique is more of a window to your soul: a pathway to inner healing, self-appreciation, and growth. This may all sound a bit strange if you have never experienced her teaching, but trust me, once you give it a try you will see for yourself.

One day Michelle invited me down to the beach for a private stretch. I had been under a great deal of stress, but for that hour stretching by the ocean I was lifted into a place of peace and growth. Of love and trust. Of freedom and hope and, best of all, pure absolute focus on myself. Since then stretch has become a daily experience for me. My body is fed by Michelle's stretch techniques. I've also been using Essential Stretch for healing and injury prevention. I have had a lot of back problems and even my doctor's prescription was to stretch every day for the rest of my life. Not drugs or painkillers or even surgery—only stretch and core strengthening. For this new dimension in my life, I thank you, Michelle. It has done more for me than you will ever know.

introduction

Just over a decade ago, as I rolled out of bed each morning I was laden with aches and pains throughout my body. My roommate at the time, Cory Everson, used me as comic relief in her fitness lectures: "This is Michelle, entering the kitchen for her morning coffee," mimicking my crippled, hunched over hobble toward the coffee machine. I was an athlete and dancer who could move with amazing precision and beautiful grace— once my body was loose and warm that is. But the stresses of life were catching up to me, showing up as injuries and tightness in my body. At the time, I thought stiffness in the morning was an inherent part of aging. But something inside of me knew I need not be in pain upon waking. This inner voice knew there was a way to heal the body through movement and it was probing me to create something.

As a dancer and choreographer I understood complete freedom of movement and did not want to lose that. I yearned to dance and enjoy an active lifestyle well into my eighties, but it was looking doubtful. To be that stiff at thirty, where would I be at forty? So I began the quest to discover a way to heal my body through movement.

Much of my initial choreography was inspired by my dance and exercise physiology studies in college. The flowing movement and grounded nature of the Luigi jazz technique particularly impressed me. Luigi developed his technique as a result of a tragic accident he had in his early twenties. After being hit by a car and thrown through a storefront window, doctors told the paralyzed young dancer he would never walk again. He refused to accept this diagnosis, truly believing that he could regain all movement if he "never stopped moving." His desire to dance again was more than fulfilled, as the rehab he created for himself became the foundation of a world renown jazz technique. I was inspired by Luigi's story and his famous quote "never stop moving," rang true to me. So as I developed my stretch technique, I choreographed movements that flowed, like a dance warm-up. These early stages of the technique were great for balance, strength, flexibility, and centering, and made sense for a dancer. It wasn't, however, a workout for everyone. And it didn't fully relax and cleanse the body. After teaching workshops throughout Europe, Canada, and the United States, I determined that changes needed to be made and set out to create a technique that was beneficial for everyone. This first routine required hard work, maintaining proper body alignment through difficult movements. It was all my body knew at the time, but the voice inside knew this wasn't the answer to releasing stress and healing injuries.

During these early developmental stages of Essential Stretch I began taking Science of Mind classes at the AGAPE International Center of Truth. I was looking for balance and peace and couldn't seem to find it on my own. Though my conscious spiritual journey began in my early twenties, this teaching catapulted my personal growth tremendously. It taught me the importance of releasing and letting go. I developed a deeper understanding of how physical, mental, and emotional stress contaminates the mind, body, and soul. It was necessary for me to learn all of this before my stretch technique could unfold into what it is today.

I realize this now as I live in a more calm state of being. Ten years ago my life was quite different. I was a human *do*ing rather than a human *being*. My workouts were centered around strength and endurance and my life was about getting things done. Sound familiar? Maybe you live that way today. And if you do, you're not alone. Despite the mind/body movement gracing the covers of major magazines, a majority still focus on toning and fat burning with little or no time devoted to stretching and restorative work. While I fully support cardiovascular and strength training, I strongly recommend balancing it with flexibility and relaxation. And I say relaxation separately because not all flexibility programs are relaxing or restorative. If you're constantly doing and controlling and contracting, you're restricting the natural flow of life. As you release your tight grip on life and relax, you open up for the natural flow of life, aligning with universal harmony. You may have read this concept in other books, but it is only when you test it in your own life that you will embody the concept and reach a true understanding of releasing and letting go to let life flow. I have seen many lives transform, including my own, through active relaxation. I wasn't always as flexible, peaceful, and free as I am today. And by no means am I saying that I am "there" or "perfect"—it is a continuous journey of progress, not perfection. But once I made the conscious choice to change the way I was treating my body, mind, and soul, a whole new way of life seemed to unfold. Through the process of creating Essential Stretch, I became more peaceful in all aspects of my life. Through consistent practice of Essential Stretch I found myself and my clients developing greater personal power, clarity, and focus resulting in many positive changes.

I am grateful for the choice I made in my early thirties and hope to inspire you to make positive choices too. I believe that in our human experience we're given the precious instruments of mind, body, and soul. We're given immense power over how these instruments will be used, neglected, or perhaps even abused. How you treat your body is your choice. How you manage your mind is your choice. How you serve your soul is also your choice. As human beings, we make choices every day that either greatly benefit us or take their toll on our lives.

So ask yourself this question: Are your daily decisions serving you well? Today is a new day. You have a fresh opportunity to become aware of what your decisions are doing for you and how to make better, wiser choices for the rest of your life.

Essential Stretch is about discovering yourself. It is not a miraculous answer to problems. It is simply a tool to guide you back to a place of wholeness where your mind, body, and soul are working together in harmony. Don't be overly concerned about goals or final results. This is your personal journey and it is the *process* that strengthens your mind/body/soul connection.

Living a blissful life is within arm's reach. We are each on our own unique path and carry our own personal issues and distinct stresses. The good news is that Essential Stretch allows you to work at your own pace. It is designed to work on the body as a whole entity, so your individual needs will be addressed as each of you benefit in your own way. If you're ready to make a commitment to yourself, read on.

It is your choice.

"In an industry cluttered with fraudulent claims, zealous marketers, money-hungry opportunists, misinformed 'experts,' and most importantly sellers who can't represent their work, it has been a relief meeting and working with someone who is so full of truth. Michelle has combined experience, reason, and intuition to develop this technique. Her technique has helped me stretch areas of my body that I have unsuccessfully been able to through yoga and personal trainers. I highly recommend Michelle's technique to everyone."—ARNEL LINDGREN

essential stretch

PART ONE

the philosophy of Essential Stretch

" 'Under pressure' . . . Somebody famous once sang that at the top of his lungs. And he was right. We are, all of us, assaulted by a daily barrage from a world grown suddenly faster . . . More dangerous . . . More overwhelming. How do you cope? What can you do to change the way the environment is hitting you day by day? Well, by changing how you react to it day by day. How you live in it. How you stretch, move and breathe in it. What if there was a technique that actually taught you a better way to flow through your life? Whether you're a star athlete, a housewife or husband who's somehow melded with the sofa. If you've opened this book—you've found it."—JERRY DIXON

ONE *the basics of Essential Stretch*

"He who knows others is wise.

He who knows himself is enlightened."—LAO-TZU

Essential Stretch is a simple movement technique. Anyone can do it—no matter what your age or fitness level—and everyone can benefit from it, even super-fit athletes and dancers. Unfortunately, when it comes to exercise programs, stretch has been placed on the back burner, or relegated to the category of exercise for the elderly. But research reveals that stretching is often the missing link in successful exercise programs. As you will see, it is becoming apparent that it may be the missing link in our lives.

the downside of ditching stretch

Do you avoid stretching? Are you the one who skips the stretch portion of a workout? Are you afraid to find out how stiff and inflexible you've become over the years? Or do you not consider it valuable enough to invest time in it? Maybe you think, like most people, that valuable workout time should be devoted to fat burning or muscle toning. Many people think the purpose of stretching is just to become flexible and do not see the bounty of benefits beyond that.

Whatever the excuse may be, avoiding stretching or something similar can put us in a position of ignorance and vulnerability regarding our health, and can keep us from being open to the natural flow of life. The more open we are, the easier we receive divine guidance pointing us in the direction of a more harmonious and peaceful way of life.

One caveat: From a physical standpoint, although stretching bears great rewards, it cannot stand alone to get you in top condition. You will still need to incorporate cardiovascular and strength training into your program. Whether you choose hiking, cycling, swimming, or dance for cardio, with muscle toning on your own or in a class, pick types of exercise that give you variety and stimulate your mind. If you receive tremendous joy from working out on the StairMaster then indulge in that. Don't pick an exercise that seems like drudgery. When you complement these programs with your Essential Stretch practice, you'll look forward to exercise because your body will feel better. But remember, your body needs all three types of exercise to function with maximum efficiency.

purpose

Essential Stretch provides two major things that many people need to reach their full potential: a simple way to undo stresses of all kinds and a link between the mind, body, and soul. When we are connected to ourselves we are better able to come from a place of wholeness where our mind, body, and soul are working in harmony. Essential Stretch is designed to cleanse the body and quiet the mind, to help us rediscover our natural balance, peace, and clarity. Much like the great Eastern forms of exercise such as yoga, tai chi, and even some martial arts, Essential Stretch is grounded in achieving harmony throughout our entire system. Although many of the breathing and mind/body focus techniques philosophically parallel yoga, the physical approach and rewards are quite different.

HOW DOES ESSENTIAL STRETCH DIFFER FROM OTHER FORMS OF STRETCH AND MIND/BODY PRACTICES?

There are five characteristics unique to Essential Stretch that set it apart from other forms of mind/body exercise such as yoga, tai chi, pilates, and other forms of stretch.

Expanded Range of Motion

The range of motion practiced in Essential Stretch is quite different from other forms of stretch and yoga. Gentle stretches, called oscillations, involve movement that flows through a range of motion beyond normal stretch or yoga positions. The range takes you outside of the normal angular positions, opening up through diagonal and circular pathways surrounding your body. This is why Essential Stretch opens you up to greater possibilities in your freedom of movement. In fact, many dancers have used this technique to improve their dance capabilities, including myself. Oscillations are like a slow dance of the muscles opening new pathways of mind/body kinesthetic awareness.

Personal Range of Motion (PROM)

Essential stretch allows you to work within your PROM. You are given the choreography or pattern of a stretch, but are not expected to push yourself to a standard position. This simply means you can accept your level and move through a range of motion that is comfortable for *you*. From that point you slowly extend a little farther through each repetition, but never beyond the point of mild discomfort. This is the Tao of expanding your range of motion gently.

Gentle and Relaxing

The emphasis is on consciously relaxing each part of the body. Where most yoga, pilates, and stretching is concerned with proper alignment and form, Essential Stretch is most concerned with letting go and relaxing. For example, in a Seated Forward Bend, instead of trying to keep your back straight and holding your neck in line with your spine, in Essential Stretch you would allow your entire torso to relax forward, letting go of the muscles in your neck and back. You would also let go of any tension in your legs, allowing your knees to bend slightly and feet to relax with no concern for pointing or flexing the toes. This allows for a better stretch, simply because your body is relaxed. Essential Stretch is designed to relax, cleanse, and stretch each and every part of the body.

Let me say that there is nothing wrong with holding your body against gravity to achieve a particular alignment—there is purpose to that as well. Those of you that are doing yoga, pilates or even other forms of stretching that put your body in those positions shouldn't worry, as you're not doing anything harmful to your body. However, be aware that if your purpose is to fully cleanse congestion and achieve complete relaxation you can not put stress on the muscles while trying to de-stress them. You can't release something if you're still holding on to it. The idea behind Essential Stretch is to release or undo all of the stress that we encounter in our life, whether it is physical, mental or emotional. To do that we must approach our workout in a way that allows us to completely release and let go.

While you are always supported in some way so the muscles being stretched can relax, some of the movements require the muscles in the waist and abdominals to contract. This does not get in the way of fully relaxing your target muscles and occurs through a phase of the stretch before you get to the full stretch position.

Using the Whole Body

Essential Stretch uses the whole body. Rather than compartmentalizing or isolating body parts, it's important to consider the whole body while stretching. Your body functions as a whole—each and every part is connected. If you have a problem in one area and it is not taken care of, it will eventually effect other areas. Likewise, as you stretch and open areas that have been blocked, you clear pathways for more energy and fluids to flow into other areas, nourishing and unblocking the rest of the body. This basic concept will help you understand why you will work through the full range of motion and allow the whole body to get involved in many of the oscillations. The oscillations in this book stretch your muscles from many different angles in just one stretch so that the entire body is engaged. Each oscillation has a primary muscle or area that we are aiming to stretch, yet all of the surrounding muscles and joints are used to encourage a stream of fluids and energy into the target area being stretched. This is another reason why you are able to indulge in a deeper stretch—you are moving beyond the traditional stretch and yoga poses.

> "Michelle has taught me how to be alive in my body, to allow my mind and body to connect freely without judgment or control. As a personal trainer I have always praised the benefits of stretch, but this approach by far is the most encompassing, challenging, and enjoyable method I have ever experienced. Since I've been doing Essential Stretch my life has transformed on many levels."—BRENDA BEARDSLEY, L.A. BASED THERAPIST AND PERSONAL TRAINER

Heart Activation

The fifth characteristic unique to Essential Stretch is activating the heart, but don't confuse this with a cardiovascular workout. Learning to consciously activate our heart energy can help in many different areas of our lives. By tapping into your heart, you will be opening a fountain of love, compassion, understanding, wisdom, creativity, bliss, and so much more. These beautiful qualities of the heart lie within each one of us. (In Chapter Three, you will learn how to align yourself with your heart, increasing the healing powers of the stretch while developing a habit of heart activation that can change your life.)

Tapping In

One of the most important reasons why you should practice Essential Stretch is to tap in. Tap in to what, you ask? Tap in to your fullest potential. If you've ever read a book or article about the mind/body connection, or if you've practiced yoga, you're probably aware of the fact that we have access to our greatest power when we are in alignment with our inner self and are fully aware in the present moment. To achieve that state of being isn't necessarily easy. We have daily distractions. We have mind-chatter, which can take us out of the present moment. And oftentimes we have tightness in our bodies that resists our openness to life.

How do we rid ourselves of the mind-pollution that blocks our ability to access inner strength and power? Oftentimes, when we try to focus inward to tap into that inner power, we meet resistance. Sometimes there's too much going on in our heads and we can't seem to relax our bodies. Essential Stretch is an active act of relaxation that helps us consciously release mind-chatter and body constriction. The gentle, flowing movements encourage the body to relax and open, creating space for the natural flow of energy. By bringing attention to your body and its movement, you become completely aware of your moment-to-moment thoughts, feelings, and sensations. This is called being mindful and will help you appreciate every aspect of your experience. Practicing mindfulness brings balance and harmony to all facets of our lives.

Essential Stretch will help you develop this positive habit of mindfulness. It is a tool that can actually change the way we live. It helps us fine-tune our ability to focus and when we learn to focus we are better able to access our creativity and productivity. You will become more grounded in your daily activities, thus gaining control over your life.

"After many years of dancing and performing, I have learned that the most important way to activate my mind, body, and spirit is through stretch. It is essential to creating unity and harmony within. This alone for me is the key to clear concentration. This fact does not apply to humans alone. Watch any animal awaken from slumber. The beauty of the stretch is evident instantly as it replenishes the nourishment one needs to survive. Stretching is your body breathing . . . period."—ERIC RED, DANCER/SINGER

PART TWO

the blessings of Essential Stretch

The blessings of Essential Stretch are endless. Practicing it on a regular basis will benefit your mind, body, soul, and ultimately, your life. Consistency is key however, since the benefits are cumulative. Whether you are interested in taming tension or injury prevention, your results will directly reflect your devotion to your practice, but you don't have to be a fanatic to achieve results. A little stretch each day goes a long way. On the surface, Essential Stretching makes you feel good and helps your body function better. Beyond that you open yourself up to unlimited possibilities!

TWO *enhance your quality of life*

"The combination of movement and stillness enables you to unleash your creativity in all directions—wherever the power of your attention takes you."—DEEPAK CHOPRA

it clears clutter

Over the years your body has been used as a receptacle for everything good and bad in your life. Food choices, health habits, environmental factors, and emotions are reflected in the state of your body. Sounds like your body is a dumping ground, doesn't it? Well, ingested by mouth or otherwise, it's not far from the truth.

Throughout our body is an amazing network of communication. Whether information is transmitted through the circulatory system, the nervous system, the endocrine system, the lymphatic system, or even through the energetic pathways, each cell in our body is somehow connected. Our body functions best when these pathways are clear. Nutrients must be delivered to every cell throughout our body, toxins and waste must be flushed out, messages must be transmitted from our brain to our muscles—the important pipelines of communication throughout our being is a long list. Problems arise when these pathways become congested from a sedentary lifestyle, poor food choices, drugs, alcohol, the air we breathe, and the physical, mental, and emotional stress we experience.

Essential Stretch provides a cleansing effect that flushes your system. While stretching cannot completely cleanse the body, it does stimulate the flow of energy and fluids. The increased circulation you'll derive from stretch has a wakening effect, helping you to feel more alive in your body. Stretching the body through various poses also promotes better drainage of the lymphatic vessels, the body's waste-removal system.[1]

your fluids will flow

There are many water-based liquids throughout the body, which I refer to as fluids throughout this book. Fluids provide a medium for transportation for all bodily functions. Every cell in our body needs to receive oxygen and nutrients and to discard waste. The movements of Essential Stretch increase the circulation of fluid to meet cellular needs.

> "It is vital for health and longevity to stretch every day. The human body is 78 percent water. Most of that fluid is found in the blood vessels, muscles, lymph, and skin organs. A strong pumping heart is essential to move the fluid that courses through our arteries and veins. The heart, however, cannot move the majority of the fluid that is stored in the muscles, lymph, and connective tissues. It is only by regularly stretching that the waste collected in the fluid of our bodily tissues may be moved into the bloodstream. Essentially, stretching is a great way to give the body a regular flush!"—RICHARD DEANDREA, M.D., N.D.

Stretching also elongates cells that are rigid or inflamed, allowing fluids to pass through and cells to receive nourishment and get rid of their waste. On a larger scale, many of the stretches massage the internal organs as well as the lymphatic system, forcing secretion of toxins and waste to be carried through the body's sea of liquids.

your qi will flow

No, that isn't a typo. Qi (pronounced chee) is a word derived from ancient Taoist manuscripts, which theorize that this subtle and formless energy is the vital life force that sustains all living things.[2] If you've been raised by the principles guiding Western civilization, this concept of energy may seem foreign and abstract. After all, qi is invisible. Yet for centuries this life force has been a central focus in Eastern medical philosophies and many different religious philosophies. In the view of Taoist philosophers, this energy permeates the human organism, making it a vast energetic network. Modern-day science and theoretical physics have only recently discovered that our bodies and minds are basically fields of energy that vibrate and move at different rates and in different ways.[3]

To enjoy optimal health, we want to stay open for this vital energy to flow through our bodies clearly and effortlessly. Qi is the underlying force of life. Every organ, action, and function of our being is driven by this vital energy, and it must be able to flow freely to maintain harmony in our systems.

Wilhelm Reich, the Austrian psychoanalyst, referred to qi as "orgone," the universal life force emanating from all organic material. He believed that one's physical and emotional well-being depends on the unobstructed flow of energy in the body.[4] When we are blocked mentally, physically, or emotionally, energy can get stuck or coagulate. This blocking of the free flow of energy causes dis-ease (or disease) in our systems. Conditions ranging from rigid character attitudes, to stiffness, tension, and pain are all possible results from the hindrance of energy flow. Energy flow can be interrupted by mechanical repetition, unnatural and painful action, one-speed compartmentalized movement, and the figurative dismemberment of body from mind and spirit.[5]

Essential Stretch encourages the flow of qi throughout our entire system. The fluid movements and wide range of motion enhance energy flow and clear pathways, which prevents obstruction. The mind/body/spirit connection also opens up energetic communication and prevents the interruption of energy flow throughout our being.

Now, just so you fully understand, stretching itself is not what expands your consciousness. It is the process that opens you up and connects you with your inner self so that *you* can do the expanding. As we stretch and relax, we open ourselves up for the natural flow of qi.

you'll feel good all over

It doesn't take a rocket scientist to figure this one out. When you stretch, you nurture your body and that makes you feel good! First, the gentle movement encourages the flow of synovial fluid into the joints for cushioning. Second, since your mind and body are actively involved in the stretch, your results are longer lasting, so you feel good longer. Third, when we lighten our load of manifest stress we feel more comfortable and lighter in our bodies.

When you stretch, certain "stretch receptors" located in and next to your muscles tell your brain that you're relaxed and feel good. The brain responds by sending chemicals of well-being (such as endorphines and serotonin) to the muscles and the nervous system. Therefore, stretching reinforces positive moods.[6]

you'll move like a pro (or a bit more like one)

Are you the one in the aerobics class always two steps behind? Agility is the ability to move quickly and easily like a skilled dancer. Do you stand on the sidelines of a funk aerobics class claiming to have two left feet? Coordination is when all the individual parts work together harmoniously, usually to achieve specific movement. Do you avoid step aerobics because you're afraid you'll trip on the step? Movement efficiency is when you are able to produce a desired movement effectively, without waste of time or energy. To be a good athlete, dancer, or even a skilled weekend warrior, you need to develop decent agility, coordination, and movement efficiency. All require good muscle-to-muscle and brain-to-muscle communication. Stretching helps to clear the lines of communication throughout the entire system so messages travel clearly and quickly. The cross-link communication in the muscles is more direct, with less collagenous fibers to create stiffness and obstructions. Stretching stimulates and regulates the nervous system and increases the effectiveness of mind/body communication. You will develop more control over your body—possibly in ways you never even imagined. Your movement can become freer, easier, and more precise, as it opens up pathways to enhance your spatial awareness and allows your body to move with greater coordination and grace.

standing tall

Maintaining good posture is essential to health and longevity. Practicing good posture can help you prevent misalignment problems. Most people think of good posture as a reflection of balanced strength and proper alignment. True, but tense muscles also impact posture. If you tense your back to maintain perfect alignment, you may look great but your body inevitably suffers because tight muscles can cause the body to become off balance and out of alignment. The key to good posture with longevity is to create balance in your muscle strength, muscular flexibility, and relaxability. Excellent and relaxed posture is essential for the natural flow of qi throughout your body.

Poor posture can set you up for long-term health problems—aches and pains and premature aging. Think about how much older you look when you slump. And how you feel when your body is stiff as a board upon waking in the morning. If you're in pain, do you get a restful sleep? Notice the extra effort it requires to move a stiff body.

better sex

Tension and anxiety can put a huge damper on your sexual enjoyment and ability to perform. Ken Goldberg, M.D., explains, "Performance anxiety is exceedingly common. Although roughly 85 percent of erection problems have some physical basis, problems in a relationship or even job stress can cause the body to overproduce erection-snuffing chemicals. It's simply not possible to separate the biological side from the emotional side."[7]

Experts believe that psychological factors including stress, anxiety, guilt, depression, low self-esteem, and fear of sexual failure are associated with more than 80 percent of cases of impotence, usually as secondary reactions to underlying physical causes.[8] Though some cases are more complicated than others, stretching helps you release tension and anxiety and can assist in preventing sexual frustration.

While mental and emotional blockages can get in the way of male performance, they also get in the way of sexual freedom in both men and women. There are no guarantees; however, stretching can definitely help you release some or all of the stuff that may be blocking you from a good orgasm.

Stretching also helps you get in touch with yourself on a deeper level and increases your body awareness. Physically, a clear, stretched body has better means of mind/body communication. In addition, it is possible that since stretching helps you feel more comfortable with yourself and your body it can make you feel sexually freer.

waist away

You think you may have a six-pack underneath that beer belly? You won't know unless you lose the adipose tissue surrounding it. (And you may have to lose the beer to gain the six-pack.) But if that's your goal, stretch should be part of your program. Although Essential Stretch was not created for the purpose of improving physical appearance, it does benefit your overall look and particularly tones the waist and abdominals. Certain oscillations trim the waistline by stretching it in one direction and strengthening it in the other direction. This is a very safe and effective way to work your waist, since you are only using your own body weight and gently moving into and out of the positions. Additionally, most of the movement is initiated from your center, and you maintain your balance through a continual connection to your center.

the missing ingredient to weight loss

Are you one of those people who spends countless hours on cardiovascular and weight training and still struggles to lose those last five pounds? You don't have to pound your body or sweat like a pig to get lean. In fact, for longer lasting results, your missing ingredient may be just the opposite—stretching. As you work out you put physical stress on your body to strengthen your muscles. In that process your body can become tight and somewhat constricted. Treating your body to a nurturing stretch elongates and opens up your muscles to receive oxygen and blood-nutrients and to eliminate waste. This helps keep your muscles balanced, strong, and healthy. Stretching regularly also helps clear blockages in problem areas, facilitating cleansing and nourishing of those areas, which eventually helps balance the entire system.

Even if you're not a workout buff, you could have stress factors or a sedentary lifestyle working against your weight loss. On an energetic level stress manifests in our bodies, coagulating energy and blocking the optimal functioning of our systems. Those of you who are stuck in the office all day or choose to be a couch potato face the same issues. As former Miss Olympia Cory Everson explained in her book *Life Balance*, "Stress causes the body to respond less effectively to good diet, training, and health efforts. It diminishes the immune system and the emotions and even encourages the body to become better at fat storage!" To that end, many people overeat and make unhealthy choices when they are emotionally stressed. Practicing Essential Stretch regularly will relieve stress and help you become more in touch with your body, giving you a new sense of peace and possibly a calm approach to eating. Eventually your natural instincts to take good care of your body will emerge and emotional eating will be a thing of the past.

enhance clarity, concentration, and creativity

"Relaxation and concentration are intertwined; one cannot relax the muscles of the toe if he cannot focus the mind's attention to that part of the body," Dr. Arya, author of *Superconscious Meditation*, explains. A tense person cannot concentrate, and a truly concentrated mind can be achieved only if you are relaxed. Concentration is the direction and control of energy. Energy locked in maintaining a physical state of tension/stress is not available for our conscious direction.[9]

Essential Stretching helps bring your mind into an alpha state, a state of conscious balance where one is awake, alert, focused, and totally relaxed. (This happens as a result of letting go of exterior distractions and surface mind-chatter by consciously relaxing the mind and body and focusing inward.) You'll notice that after an Essential Stretch workout your perception becomes very clear and creative juices flow freely.

This is a state of consciousness, sometimes called one-pointedness, or single-pointedness, where we steady our mind and practice focusing our attention on the here and now. Cultivating this kind of concentration is one way to wake up from the dream of ordinary consciousness to become more alive and more aware in our choices. This is the state of mind people look to achieve from meditation, yoga, and qi gong.

rejuvenate and slow aging down

"The bodily decrepitude presumed under the myth of aging is not inevitable. It is, by and large, both avoidable and reversible."—THOMAS HANNA

We all face the challenges of aging, and—due to our stressful lifestyles—many of us are aging quicker than we need to. Stress causes degeneration of cells and as cells become damaged they lose their ability to retain fluid and so become dehydrated. Damaged cells also have a tough time absorbing nutrients, which affects the way our entire system works. Stretch is not going to eliminate stress; however, it can change the way your body reacts to it and can save you from damaging more cells. As you relax and open pathways through stretching, the circulation of blood-nutrients and oxygen is increased. When your system flows clearly, cells regenerate and absorb nourishment more easily.

From a muscular standpoint, we are most flexible between the ages of six and twelve. Depending on our lifestyle, flexibility decreases from there. Unless we keep our muscles strong and flexible, as we age, the connective tissue inside muscles starts to shorten and become dense with collagen fibers. These fibers are strong but not flexible, and they tighten and weaken muscles. Our cross-link communication becomes congested (cross-links are the muscles' communication system) and messages sent between the muscles meet more resistance, which negatively affects our agility and coordination. Also, since we become more dehydrated as we age, our tendons and joints tend to "dry up" and carry less protective synovial fluid. As one becomes stiffer with age, simple tasks in life become more difficult.

Stretching regularly is the best preventative medicine for these dilemmas. It elongates your muscles and keeps cross-link communication more direct and clear. Oscillations help keep joints lubricated with synovial fluid and can prevent us from becoming rigid as we age. This way we have the option to stay active well into our later years.

THREE *prevent and heal adversities*

stress management

What exactly is stress? The word "stress" comes from a Latin word that means "tight." According to *The Holistic Health Handbook*, "Stress is any condition that harms the body or damages, breaks down or causes the death of few or many cells. Nobody can escape stress. Stress merely means life. It has been defined as the rate of wear and tear caused by living."[1]

It is no secret that today more than ever people are overloaded with stress of one kind or another. We live in a fast-paced society with work pressures, family issues, relationship tribulations, ego expectations, worldly matters—the list is endless. Millions are stiffening up and aging quicker than they'd like. To cope with these complaints, Americans alone consume five billion tranquilizers, five billion barbiturates, three billion amphetamines, and sixteen thousand tons of aspirin (not including ibuprofen and acetaminophen) every year.[2]

Millions turn to alcohol and comfort food to cope. Unfortunately, none of these self-medicating methods reach the root of the problem. They only mask symptoms. No matter where stress comes from, it manifests in the body and clogs our systems if it's not alleviated. Since it accumulates slowly (even over a period of years), you may not realize the toll stress takes on the body. From the time we are babies we begin to accumulate stress: from feelings of rejection to the strain of competition, from the pain of a relationship breakup to everyday work-related tension. It can even stem from the physical stress you place on your body when working out with weights. But it's not the individual stresses that are harmful—it's the accumulation of stresses that can result in major health problems.

WHERE DOES STRESS COME FROM?

There are three types of stress: physical, mental, and emotional. Physical stress can occur from simply sitting for long periods of time. It can be brought on by everyday life, such as carrying a purse on one shoulder and putting your body off balance. It can also be the result of active, healthy pursuits such as weight lifting or jogging. If you indulge in a fitness program without stretching to rebalance muscles, you may induce tightness and create blockages in the musculoskeletal system. Sometimes it's movement that stresses the body, and other times it's inactivity, as the body becomes stagnant.

Mental stresses also impact the body. Financial pressures, marriage and relationship problems, and the inability to express yourself can all manifest as stress in the body.

Emotional stresses such as loneliness, frustration, hatred, sadness, anger, fear, and loss affect the body as well. If you believe that you're one of those rare unemotional people, does that mean you don't suffer from emotional stress? Not necessarily. In fact, if you're not allowing yourself to express your emotions, you could become "emotionally constipated." What you choose not to deal with will inevitably get pushed down and buried deep within your system, and as you continue to unconsciously bury stress it accumulates and results in tremendous tightness in your body.

HOW DOES STRESS AFFECT OUR HEALTH?

Stress is the root of much unhappiness, disharmony, sickness, and other problems. It is no secret that stress manifests in the body, and the buildup can adversely affect our health. It's bad enough having a tight upper back or feeling like you're carrying a ton of bricks on your shoulders, but when you don't take action to find the source of stress and deal with it, you set yourself up for worse health problems in the future. According to the American Institute of Stress (AIS), 43 percent of all adults suffer adverse health effects due to stress. 75 to 90 percent of all visits to primary care physicians are for stress-related complaints or disorders. Stress has been linked to all the leading causes of death, including heart disease, cancer, lung ailments, accidents, cirrhosis, and suicide. And recent research has increasingly confirmed the important role of stress in cardio-vascular disease, cancer, gastrointestinal, skin, neurologic and emotional disorders, and a host of disorders linked to immune system disturbances, ranging from the common cold and herpes, to arthritis, cancer, and AIDS.[3]

HOW CAN ESSENTIAL STRETCH ALLEVIATE STRESS?

"The concept of energy and of the flow of that energy in the human body is the core of the current explosion in healing. The healing principle is to 'balance' the energy in the body by using relaxation to counter the body's reaction to stress."—THE HOLISTIC HEALTH HANDBOOK, THE BERKELEY HOLISTIC HEALTH CENTER

We can't avoid stress because it is a part of our human life. But we can learn how to manage it so that it doesn't affect our health and happiness. By creating a state of homeostasis we can avoid the disturbance that stress would normally cause in our system. Homeostasis is our ability to maintain internal stability, regardless of stimuli that would disturb our normal condition. This, however, is easier said than done. Stretching alone is not going to help you maintain complete homeostasis, but it can help. By actively relaxing your body and quieting your mind you are creating a calm inner atmosphere. If stress does arise, your reaction is going to be less harmful and alarming to your system.

After you have worked with Essential Stretch and maybe other mind/body/spirit type work, you will most likely become more grounded and centered. This helps us deal with stress much more gracefully. When we move from our center, from a place of peace and clarity, we are less likely to get confused and fly off the handle. We are more likely to rise above tough situations and find solutions rather than dwell on the problem itself.

Essential Stretch not only works on relieving stress that has manifested in the body, but also creates a state of being that can better handle stressful situations. Stress is not 100 percent of the problem. It is how we handle stress that determines its affects on our body and our health. Much of how we react to stress depends on how we have learned to relax. Just as you would have to train your body to run a mile in less than eight minutes, you have to train your body to relax. Relaxation can counter the body's reaction to stress. Therefore, by practicing Essential Stretch relaxation techniques you can help prevent many stress-related conditions and diseases.

"I am a type-A personality with a very demanding job. I go a million miles an hour all day and find it very hard to relax. Essential Stretch is the catalyst I need to slow down. Within the first five minutes of class, I have slowed down my heart rate, started focusing on my breath, and can feel the muscles in my body releasing tension. After thirty minutes, I am in a deep state of relaxation and my stresses from the day start to melt away. At the completion of the class, I leave in a state of mindfulness that renders me invulnerable to the pressures of life. I highly recommend Essential Stretch to everyone of all levels. Michelle's style is gentle and uplifting, and you will look forward to coming back to her class again and again."
—ALANA ROSS, TECHNOLOGY SYSTEMS ANALYST, LOS ANGELES, CA

CAN YOU BE STRESSED WITHOUT REALIZING IT?

Yes. When you're not in tune with your body, you can be numb to the stress that is within. A 1997 Duke University study revealed that only a minority of heart patients experienced pain. Even though they were in serious danger of a heart attack, they were completely unaware that a buildup of stress was affecting their hearts. Their awareness of their bodies was so diminished that they couldn't feel what was happening.[3] When pathways throughout your body are blocked, it obstructs your sensitivity and feeling. When the cells throughout your muscles and nerves are not getting the proper nutrition because pathways are clogged, they are not able to work efficiently.

Do you walk around feeling connected to your body with complete awareness of how your body feels? Or does your head feel separate from your body? Or do you ignore your body? Are you numb from the neck down?

Try this simple exercise:
Sit down and feel your feet on the ground.
Notice how your legs feel, and how your butt feels on the surface it's resting on.
Is your back straight or are you hunching over?
How are you breathing? Is it shallow? Deep?
Do you have any tension in your neck, trapezius, or upper back?
Do you have any pain anywhere in your body?
Are you holding any tension in your face?

Answer these questions honestly, but don't beat yourself up about them, just analyze your physical feelings. When was the last time you did that? Have you ever thought about how your body actually felt?

Now if you haven't paid much attention to your body before now, don't start judging yourself and regretting the way you've lived. That was your path up until now. Simply accept that fact and, though the accumulation of stress may have left a few scars, those experiences brought lessons into your life. At this point if you choose to work on releasing the scars of stress, you can do that by becoming more aware of your body through Essential Stretch.

"It takes an accumulation of stress to stiffen the body—
and takes an accumulation of stretch to cleanse it."

you'll tame tension

Temporomandibular joint syndrome (TMJ), headaches, backaches, nervous system disorders, kinks, stomach spasms, and constipation are just a few examples of illnesses often caused by physical and emotional tension. The way we react to physical, mental, and emotional stresses can cause disturbances in our body. Instead of a balanced, peaceful, and harmonious vessel, our body becomes tight and anxiety-ridden. These obstructions in our muscular system can affect everything from our movement efficiency to our mood. When our bodies feel stiff and out of sorts, we can become irritable and less creative. It takes time to work through and completely release tension, but with consistent Essential Stretching you can reduce and oftentimes completely eliminate symptoms.

Stretching inspires your muscles to "progressively relax." It reduces the amount of electrical firing inside the muscle, which keeps the muscle tight. This does not change the density of the muscle tissue, so no worries about losing firmness in your muscles. What it *does* do is release tension in the muscle, which lengthens and unwinds knots and congestion. This clears and opens the muscle tissue, allowing it to easily absorb nutrients and dispose of waste products.

you'll prevent injuries

Injuries often occur because the body is overly tight in one area, which causes misalignment. When the body is out of alignment it compensates in an attempt to rebalance itself. Rather than rebalancing, however, it actually manipulates other areas into unnatural states. This often results in overuse or chronic injuries. If the tightness is not corrected (stretched out), problems may gradually move on to other body parts and worsen. By stretching the entire body and easing tight areas you can rediscover your natural balance and prevent injuries from creeping up on you.

Stretching regularly improves circulation, sending blood-nutrients to your muscles and joints, which helps keep your muscles and connective tissues more elastic and less likely to get injured. Stretching also lubricates your joints with synovial fluid, which provides extra cushioning to the joints (so you can safely slide into home plate!), creating more freedom of movement and protecting the joints from injury. Stretching also helps keep the lines of communication (the cross-links) clearer and therefore aids in more efficient muscular contraction and reaction.

Essential Stretch helps prevent acute injuries. As you increase your range of motion, you lower your risk of over-extending yourself. So you can go out and play ball or take an aerobics class without fear of pulling something. It also improves your kinesthetic awareness and increases your coordination, agility, and flexibility—all factors that help prevent injuries.

For those of you who enjoy sports or other recreational activities, to prevent injuries give yourself a warm-up and stretch before your activity and a decent amount of time to stretch and undo after your activity. You need to lengthen those muscles you've tightened during your activity to rebalance your body. The five-minute cooldown that most people do is hardly sufficient. It usually takes a minimum of twenty minutes to stretch everything, but that depends on the workout and the individual. You'll learn how to listen to your body and do what feels right to you.

By using stretch in your warm-up and cooldown you can also prevent soreness and injuries. Stretching in the warm-up prepares your body for the activity that follows. The cooldown lengthens the muscles that have been tightened during the workout, preventing the body from holding on to the tightness and creating imbalances.

quit sounding like a whoopee cushion

Ever felt bloated, even when you haven't eaten that much? Maybe you become more aware of some abdominal distension when you try and suck in your stomach or, worse yet, when you can't button your pants. Those uncomfortable extra inches can sometimes be the result of constipation or excess air in the intestines. Once again, stress shows up as a main offender. Deep breathing and stretch can help to decrease stress and lessen these symptoms. Furthermore, some of the movements massage internal organs helping to move out excess air and bring more qi and blood-nutrients into those areas. Although stretching can help, don't rely totally on stretching for alleviating intestinal disorders.

headaches

There are three main types of headaches: tension, migraine, and sinus. Tension headaches are the most common and are usually caused by physical, mental, or emotional stress. Tightness in the neck and shoulders seems to be the most direct cause and can be caused by anything from hours of typing, to carrying around a baby, to stressful deadlines at work. With the accumulation of stress, the muscles get tighter and can create trigger points, which are spots where the muscles have become extremely irritated. Myofascial trigger points in any of the muscles of the neck and shoulders can trigger pain in the head, behind the eyes, at the base of the skull, and in the back or side of the head, or they can create that "tight band" feeling around the head.[4] Headaches initiated by tension can be prevented and oftentimes alleviated by stretching the muscles in the neck and shoulder area.

Since migraines are vascular in nature, their causes are usually more complicated than those of tension headaches. However, neck and shoulder tension can produce an environment where migraines are triggered more readily and may make them more severe. During a migraine, the brain becomes engorged with blood and the blood needs somewhere to go to bring relief. If the muscles in the neck and shoulders are tight, they constrict the blood's circulation. Increasing flexibility in the neck and shoulders can help to reduce the frequency, duration, and/or intensity of a migraine.

backaches

Billions of dollars are spent each year on health care for backaches (particularly lower back pain). The irony is that lower back pain can be prevented with exercise and stretching. Inactivity and improper movement and posture are main factors that cause and aggravate this condition. For example: If you sit for long periods of time without stretching you set yourself up for the possibility of lower back pain. The position of sitting shortens the muscles surrounding and attached to the lower back, which creates muscle imbalances and tends to pull or strain the lower back. Many nerves run through the lower back and pelvic area, so tight muscles also restrict nerve function. Without regular release and rebalance these muscles get tighter with time and can develop into chronic tension—at that point, it doesn't take much to throw out your back.

As muscles become tighter they can create pressure on the joints, vertebrae, and spinal nerves, sending pain down the leg and other areas of the body. Oftentimes surgery, medication, or bed rest is prescribed, but these do not treat the *cause* of the problem. The most common cause is tight muscles from inactivity, improper body mechanics, or overuse. With inactivity and bed rest, the soft tissue becomes even more stiff and inflexible, decreasing the amount of circulation necessary for healing. Many authorities believe that bed rest is actually the worst treatment: According to the authors of the *British Clinical Guidelines for the Management of Acute Back Pain*, "For acute or recurrent low back pain with or without referred leg pain, bed rest from two to seven days is worse than placebo or ordinary activity." Gordon Waddell, M.D., author of a recent systematic review on bed rest as treatment for back pain says, "Traditional management of back pain by rest is now discredited . . . we no longer use bed rest to treat any other musculoskeletal condition." You can treat the cause or prevent the condition by stretching the muscles of the back, hips, hip flexors, glutes, and hamstrings regularly. It also helps to strengthen the abdominals. No painkiller in the world can actually fix the cause of this problem. Stretching can.[5]

decrease menstrual cramping and back pain

During your cycle when your lower back and stomach are in turmoil, would you do anything to get rid of this aggravation? Most women would agree that not only is it physically irritating, but it also adds to mood swings during this time of the month. Most menstrual pain is due to inflammation and stuck energy, which muscles react to by cramping up. The muscles in the stomach, lower back, hips, and hip flexors are the main offenders. There are many stretches that can drastically reduce cramping through these areas. Furthermore, stretching can help reduce inflammation by increasing your circulation. Relief may sometimes only be temporary, but it can help you through those uncomfortable stages.

ease arthritis

Arthritis is an umbrella term for over one hundred different conditions that affect the joints. Osteoarthritis and rheumatoid arthritis are the most common (osteoarthritis more so, affecting approximately sixteen million Americans); both can be tricky and confusing conditions. Because movement is oftentimes painful for arthritic patients, many stop moving and adopt a sedentary lifestyle, which only worsens the condition. Inactivity creates more stiffness in affected joints as well as other areas of the body. Inactivity often leads to weight gain, which also aggravates the condition. Depending on the severity of the condition, medication or specific nutrition may be necessary in the treatment of arthritis, but the most important thing you can do to help yourself is exercise. Smooth forms of exercise that are easier on the joints are recommended, such as swimming, walking, stretching, and biking. Essential Stretch's gentle nature is a perfect type of movement for arthritis sufferers.

FOUR *catapult personal growth*

boost your emotional well-being

Fitness programs exploded in the 80s and 90s, with people like Jane Fonda and Dr. Ken Cooper leading the way to better health. Despite the good intentions of the fitness movement, the emphasis placed on peak performance and body image went awry. Fitness fanatics abounded, concentrating more on excessive speed, obsessive dieting, and an unrealistic body image than nurturing the mind, body, and soul. The trends seemed to emphasize a disconnected, impractical, unattainable vision of human life. Self-appreciation was lost. The extreme was prized.

Not to blame the fitness movement for all of our problems, but fitness during this time brought about a lot of body self-consciousness. People of all ages carry the burden and negative energy of self-judgment and self-condemnation. Oftentimes this energy alone is enough to block you from the very thing you set out to do in the first place—get healthier and/or lose weight. The irony of the fitness movement is that the focus on the exterior has hidden the truth of the interior and we've lost sight of what's really healthy. When we are truly connected to our inner self we instinctively know what is right for our mind, body, and soul and make choices that benefit us mentally, physically, and emotionally. Essential Stretch helps you reconnect with your inner self and live from a space of wholeness, allowing you to dance through life free of self-judgment and self-condemnation.

active relaxation

When you are in the driver's seat you play an active role in getting to your destination. When you are the passenger, you're not actively involved (unless you are the navigator), so you are passive. As a driver you would tend to remember the direction you're driving; a passenger can tune out and not recall how he got from one point to another.

Essential Stretch is an active form of relaxation. When your mind and body are active in the process of relaxing you develop greater muscle memory and can maintain that state of relaxation or homeostasis longer. So if you have the choice—and you do— be your own driver.

> One of my students, Kevin Kingsbury, a computer systems administrator, stretches at his desk. He says, "It's like a breath of fresh air that eases the tension right away. It helps me relax and not hold on to things that would normally bother me throughout the day. Through stretching, I've discovered that I hold most of my tension in my neck and upper back. So I do the Neck and Upper Back Rolls at my desk at least three times a day— everyday!"

As you work with Essential Stretch and are able to bridge the gap between your thinking mind and feeling body, you create a flow that moves energy through blockages.

This can cleanse some of the emotional rubbish stuck in the body, which oftentimes is the root of many problems. By doing this we lower the recurrence rate of these issues.

Ultimately, you are the only one who can heal yourself. Things like Essential Stretch, counseling, and massage are simply tools to help you along your path. Our soul is on a journey to grow, develop, and unfold into greater enlightenment. Peeling away the layers of stress is a process that takes attention and intention. Learning to tame our ego and reconnect our mind, body, and soul is not easy, but it is key. By taking an active role in this process you can catapult your soul to another level. By becoming more aware and cleansing ourselves we can rise above the things that keep us down.

self-awareness

Have you ever caught a glimpse of yourself in a window and noticed your face was stern with tension? Have you ever looked at a photo of yourself and been surprised to see your shoulders were hunching? Or your belly was protruding? Essential Stretching helps us become more aware of ourselves. The technique trains you to become an observant commander of your body. You'll be able to catch yourself in poor posture and readily correct it because you'll become acutely aware of what your body is doing at all times. When we become more sensitive to how we feel in different areas of our body, we become more cognizant of our health. Learning where we hold tension and anxiety and where we may be out of alignment can guide us to stretch and cleanse those areas, helping to prevent health problems. As we learned in Chapter One, tightness may stem from physical, mental, and emotional sources, but in the end it is all energy. No matter what causes energy to become stuck, creating stiffness or blockages, it must still be untangled, flushed, or cleared. As the process of stretching helps us become more aware of our bodies, this increased awareness, in turn, gives us the knowledge of where we need to focus our stretching and conscious relaxation. Remember, "Energy flows where your attention goes,"—this is the springboard to healing.

On a deeper level, as we become more sensitive, we become more aware of our triggers or sensitive issues that ignite tension in our bodies. We call these our stressors. By learning to identify our stressors we can actively change our reaction and/or counter the stress with on-the-spot active relaxation. All of this is dependent on awareness!

relax your mind

While you're reading this book, what else is on your mind? If you're like most people, you probably have several things floating through your mind during the course of your reading. Our minds are constantly busy, replaying bits of the past and/or planning or worrying about the future. If your mind isn't in the present moment, you're missing out on the fullness of life. If you're hanging on to something from the past, or worrying about something in the future, you're not enjoying the present. This is a great chance for you to say STOP! Give your mind a break. Just be right where you are in the stretch, be in your body—not in your head. This will be very relaxing for your mind, and the more time to relax you give your mind, the easier it is to get in touch with your true self. Our ego tends to get in the way of our conscious connection to our true self, our essence. By calming our mind we clear the space, opening up to be in the present moment and receive divine guidance. We see much more clearly when we are not bogged down by the weight of our own mind. We're better able to see the truth. The time we take to quiet our mind is invaluable, as it revitalizes our connection with our infinite source and points us in the direction of our highest good.

"Essential Stretch relaxes me. It feels like I release blocked up energy, because after I stretch I feel open and calm."—NEALIE NISSINOFF, ART DIRECTOR, CALIFORNIA

emotional release

Because the attention of Essential Stretch is directed inward and you connect with various psychophysical aspects of yourself, different emotions can arise during the process. If you're interested in personal growth this is a good thing. Suppressed emotions that are buried in our muscles and joints basically form coagulated energy. Whether it is suppressed anger, resentment, or sadness, the stress of the emotion causes cells to tighten and contract. As you do things to elongate—like stretch—you open the space for these old emotions to release. As you slowly move through oscillations, you encourage the flushing of these issues. It is important to stay in your body and feel. Stay out of your head and out of judgment. Allow yourself to be with the process without intellectualizing it. By staying in your body you can avoid the ego stepping in and pushing that emotion back down. It may be emotionally uncomfortable—which is why the ego tries to step in—yet after it passes, the clearing is well worth the small amount of discomfort.

"I was going through a breakup from a five-year relationship with my boyfriend. A tremendous amount of anxiety, fear, and resentment were blocking my clear vision and beginning to run my life into the ground. I began taking Essential Stretch religiously—and literally it was like going to church for me. It made me feel so much better. It helped to reduce my negative feelings and gradually changed them to positive, more peaceful feelings. I was able to get my confidence back and be happy again."—JENNY ISHAHARA, PERSONAL TRAINER AND JAPANESE INTERNATIONAL TRADE CONSULTANT

PART THREE

bringing out the power
of Essential Stretch

In this section you will learn about different tools which enhance your stretch experience. Breathing, meditation, centering, moving oscillations, and heart activation can all be employed to deepen your experience. Stretching can be a physical and very mechanical experience; however, if you take a mind/body approach and engage in each moment with complete awareness, you can elevate your experience and boost your benefits another level.

These tools will teach you to nurture your mind/body/soul relationship. Just like a relationship with a friend or loved one, if you don't communicate with that person you don't stay connected and the relationship becomes distanced. When we allow our mind/body/soul relationship to weaken, it can affect many aspects of our lives, from coordination, circulation, and productivity, to creativity, joy, and manifestation. As we strengthen this relationship and become more in touch with ourselves, it can affect everything from decision making to our sex life.

Now it may take some time to learn to incorporate these tools into your stretching, but that's okay—in the meantime you will still get results. Just know that as you are able to involve these tools more and more your rewards will multiply.

FIVE *oscillations*

Oscillations are stretches that involve motion. They are specifically choreographed to open the body for the natural flow of qi. Depending on the stretch, the movement flows either forward and back, side to side, up and down, or it rolls around in a circular motion. No matter in what direction you're flowing, much like a pendulum there is always an equality of movement—a movement and a counter movement. The range of motion in an oscillation will be different for each individual. I call this your personal range of motion (PROM), defined as the range through which you are able to move while maintaining muscular relaxation. It is important to work in your own relaxation zone so that you don't trigger your muscles to resist against the stretch—the stretch reflex. The stretch reflex is your muscle's response to pain. When you stretch beyond the point of mild discomfort, your muscles respond by tightening or gripping against the stretch. In a form of movement where the goal is to achieve relaxation and opening, this doesn't work. Essential Stretch is designed to take the pain out of stretching so that relaxing and opening become easier and more comfortable.

Oscillations have a primary muscle or area which is being targeted, yet all of the surrounding muscles and joints become involved through the motion. This not only stretches more of the body, but also helps to increase the stream of fluids and energy into the target area. The choreography of the slow, fluid movement promotes an increase in energy flow and opening of the body. It is not necessary to push yourself to get quicker results. Be gentle with your oscillations and poses and you will achieve healthy and long-lasting results. You do not want to go beyond the point of mild discomfort—the motto here is *"No pain, more gain."*

In Part Four you will learn specific oscillations with illustrations and instructions. Although the illustrations are shown in a sequence of still photos, you want to maintain continuous fluid movement throughout the entire stretch. The rate that you move through the oscillations is up to you; however, slower is better when you are trying to achieve mind/body connection. Sometimes it's easier to start faster to get the energy rolling and loosen the body, then gradually slow down to a pace where you can really connect. Just be aware that if you do decide to move through a stretch quickly, keep it gentle and graceful and make sure you don't bounce into the stretch.

Oscillations are generally repeated several times. The goal is to go a little bit farther into the stretch through each repetition. Over time the knots and coagulated energy will loosen and eventually dissipate. This allows you to move deeper into the stretch, as the muscles and energy pathways become clearer.

oscillation variations

While oscillations bring us through a wide range of motion, they help us become aware of our bodies and specific areas that may need extra attention. This is where the stretch becomes even more personal. The idea here is to work on your own blocks by tuning in and listening to your body. These techniques help to sharpen mind/body communication. Once you have identified an area that feels blocked or tight, try applying the following techniques.

SHORT RANGE ROLL

This technique is unique to Essential Stretch and can also be utilized during many different oscillations; however, it's a little easier with positions where your weight is fully supported, as in sitting or lying-down positions. This particular technique allows you to hone in on a specific area and massage the muscle with movement. Begin by executing the oscillation a few times, observing your body through the entire movement.

Once you have identified the areas of tightness, move through the oscillation to the first area. Put all of your attention into that area. Then very gently and slowly roll back and forth through the congestion. The object is to flush energy into the blocked area with a short range of motion roll, like a rolling pin on a piece of dough. Each time you roll across the dough it smoothes out and lengthens a little bit more; each time you roll across the tightness in the muscle, it lengthens and opens up a little bit more. The gentle movement characteristic of this technique also helps you to avoid the stretch reflex. Just as you get to the point where it would become painful you roll right out of it.

VISUALIZATION

These techniques can be used with any oscillation. Perform the oscillation a few times all the way through, observing how your body feels through each part. When you're ready to go deeper, as you move through the range of the stretch when you feel a knot or tightness, gently stop and surrender into that space. Bring all of your attention and focus into that space. Once you are fully connected with that area, try one of the following visualization techniques:

Send cleansing breath: As you inhale, visualize bringing fresh, clean oxygen directly into the congested area. Visualize this air gently washing through the clutter, dissolving the congestion. As you exhale, visualize your breath carrying out the toxins. Repeat this several times, until you feel you have released as much as you can at this time.

Send a mind/body message: Your mind is much more powerful than you may realize. In this technique you simply tell your muscle to "release," "relax," or "let go." Intense concentration is essential in order to achieve the desired release. This one may take a bit more practice, but in the long run will be a great technique to improve mind/body teamwork.

Send heart energy: You can read more about this in the heart activation section in Chapter Seven. In this technique, first you need to focus into your heart space and stay there until you really feel connected. Once you feel you have connected with your heart energy, inhale while focusing into your heart, and as you exhale send that heart energy into the area on which you're working. This too, takes a good bit of practice, but the more you work on it the easier and more gratifying it becomes.

Send a smile: This has a similar feel to the heart activation and can be an extension of it. You can visualize sending a smile directly, or you can send the smile from your heart. Either way the smile represents joy and can be very healing to the body.

I recommend closing your eyes (if it's comfortable) for all of the above techniques. This will help you focus inward. The more you are able to focus, connect, and relax, the sooner you will feel a release in that muscle. Once you have felt a release you can either stay there and sink a little deeper, or continue to move through the range of motion until you feel the next kink or tightness and repeat the deep focus into that area. These are great techniques to practice as you're stretching by yourself because you can feel free to take as much time as you need. When your mind/body connection is really developed your body will relax like magic.

The four visualization techniques can also be used in static stretches.

static stretching

Static stretching has been used for years, and is a great way to focus on a stretch. A static stretch is a single-position, motionless stretch. Most experts would explain this method as a ten- to sixty-second hold in a single-stretch position. In Essential Stretch I do not like to use the word "hold," since it can cause people to lock into a position. In addition, to the naked eye the external position appears rigid and inactive; however, when you are stretching, the object is to lengthen the muscles, even if it's microscopic lengthening. If you're sending messages to your brain like "I must hold this position for twenty seconds," your brain is likely to cause your muscles to lock up and stay still. Once again, this is where visualization can aid in your stretching. Even though your body is not visually moving, you want to imagine your muscles gradually extending. The key is to think: relax, release, and extend!

There is also the danger of activating the stretch reflex in this type of stretching since you are in the position for more than two seconds. To avoid this, it is key to listen to your body and stay away from stretching to the point of pain. By remaining gentle with your body, you will be able to relax your muscles more; therefore, it is beneficial to take it easy and only stretch to the point of mild discomfort.

Oftentimes in Essential Stretch we weave static stretching into oscillations. This lessens the chance of the muscles and joints "locking up," as the movement promotes the surge of energy and fluids through the body. For example, we may begin the Pigeon Pose with a static stretch and breathe into the lower back and hip for about a minute, and then incorporate a Short Range Roll. Or we may begin a stretch with the movement, and once we feel the muscles have started to release, we sink into a static stretch for a moment of focus and visualization or breath work. Static stretching can be used throughout your stretch routine, just remember to continue to relax and envision elongating your muscles.

six *breath*

Breath is life. When you are born into this world your first breath signifies the fact that you are alive. When you depart, your last breath signifies the cessation of this life. All that time in between you breathe with or without your conscious awareness. Since breathing comes naturally, it is often taken for granted, unrecognized for its powerful nature. As you will experience through Essential Stretch practices, your breath can be a bridge to peace and relaxation.

Research has long supported breath as an effective stress reliever. A recent *Time* magazine article reported "Breathing exercises have been shown to decrease blood pressure and lower levels of stress hormones."[1] Many of the Eastern philosophies, such as yoga and tai chi, have known and respected the value of breath and have incorporated breathing practices into technique. Rolf Sovik, Psy.D., who did his doctoral project on the effects of breath training in the treatment of panic disorder, explains, "Practicing relaxed, diaphragmatic breathing is refreshing and restful, and creates a sense of well-being. It calms the nervous system, helps prevent psychosomatic disturbances, including panic episodes, and centers attention."[2]

Deep, relaxed belly breathing (diaphragmatic breathing) is an integral part of Essential Stretch. We utilize breath to melt deeper into a stretch, to connect one movement to the next, and to connect our mind to our body. Breath is the doorway to our heaven within, the gateway to our inner self. If your breath is shallow, tight, or constricted it is difficult to relax and reach the depths of your being. Likewise, when you experience anxiety or stress, notice how your breath becomes short or restricted. As you practice Essential Stretch and/or one of the deep breathing techniques to follow, you will find it easier to relax, calm anxiety, and effortlessly breathe deep.

Try the following practices to help you get in touch with your breath.

Echoes in the Water, or Isolated Underwater Breathing:

Lay in the bathtub with your ears under the water and listen to your breath (your nose and mouth are above the water). This helps to cut off exterior sounds and enhances your ability to hear inside of yourself. It will sound as though your breath is magnified, though it is the same volume as always, you just hear it better. You are also tapping into the vibration that your breath creates throughout your body. This is a wonderful way to connect with your breath and to learn to let your breath carry you inward. Allow your breath to flow naturally, and as you fall into deeper relaxation notice how your breath reaches further into the depths of your being.

Feeling Breath:

Lie down on your back and place your hands on your lower abdomen. Notice how your breath occurs naturally. Feel the rise and fall in your belly as you breathe. If your breath is not reaching your belly, observe the path of your inhalation and everything surrounding it, from the time it comes in through your nostrils. Notice your nasal passageways. Are they congested? As it moves down the back of your throat, is your throat constricted in any way? Is your neck tense? As it travels down into your chest and lungs, are your ribs restricting your breathing in any way? Is your chest tight? Is your belly constricting your breath? Once you are aware of the idiosyncrasies your body carries, then you can begin the healing process. Consciously relax each body part that needs it. Remember, energy flows where your attention goes, but first you must know where to put your attention. Do this as long as you would like. The goal is to reach a point where your breathing is deep (into your belly), calm, and effortless.

Complete Breath workout:

This workout will help you feel the difference between chest breathing and belly breathing (diaphragmatic breathing), and will also help open the entire breath pathway. Optimally, you want to develop your belly breathing and use that for your everyday breathing. Chest breathing is not suggested for all-day breathing. This can be done in any position; however, if you're just beginning it may be easiest to lie on your back so that your spine is straight and your body is fully supported by the earth, allowing all of your muscles to completely relax.

Step one: Breathe slowly and deeply into your belly allowing it to expand with each breath. *Repeat four times*

Step two: Breathe slowly and deeply into your chest allowing your rib cage to expand with each breath. *Repeat four times.*

Step three: Combine step one and two into one breath. Start by breathing deeply into your belly. Once your belly is completely full of air, continue to take in more air allowing your rib cage to fully expand. Exhale very slowly, emptying the air out of your rib cage first and then your stomach. Contract your belly button into your spine at the end of your exhale to expel any last bit of air. *Repeat at least four times.*

The complete breath workout can be done anytime to loosen up restriction in your breathing and to help calm stress and anxiety. This is also a great way to warm up your breath before a workout.

INCORPORATING YOUR BREATHING WHILE STRETCHING:

Those who have practiced breathing techniques through voice lessons, yoga, or other disciplines and are keenly aware of their breath may find this natural. However, since most of us take breathing for granted, it's very important to take note of the value of breathing correctly. Breath is the bridge that connects our thinking minds to our feeling bodies. It can bring us deeper into our stretch, facilitating the relaxation of our muscles.

Oftentimes, until we are comfortable with a movement or body position, we tend to tense up, take shallow breaths, or hold our breath in the process of learning something unfamiliar. This is exactly the opposite of what we want to do while stretching. Slow, deep, and complete breathing helps our mind and body to relax. It also supplies oxygen that is needed by every cell in our body, including our brain. When you breathe completely you get seven times more oxygen than when you take shallow chest breaths. When our mind, body, and breathing are relaxed, we open up to enjoy the full benefits of stretch.

Try the following techniques while you're stretching and see what works best for you.

METHOD ONE *breath awareness*

In this method you simply observe your breath, and by doing so you can learn a lot about yourself.

Is your breathing shallow or deep?

Does your breath feel constricted in any way?

Notice how your breath changes through each stretch. When a stretch gets more difficult, what happens to your breath?

Do you ever hold your breath?

Is your breathing different when you're standing as opposed to lying down?

Does your breathing change from the beginning to the end of your workout?

This method will help you to understand what you need to work on.

METHOD TWO *synchronized breath*

In this method you weave your breath into the movement of the stretch.

Before beginning the stretch take a nice deep breath.
Then as you move into the stretch, exhale. (Exhaling into the stretch encourages your muscles to relax.)
As you move away from the fully extended position you inhale again.
Then exhale into the next stretch position.

You're creating a steady rhythm with your breath and movement so that your body and breath synchronize into harmony with one another. As your body and breath work in sync with one another, the effectiveness of this partnership flourishes. This breathing technique works really well with oscillations by creating a steady flow of body and breath into and out of each position.

METHOD THREE *breath visualization*

This method increases your mind/body awareness on a deep and intricate level. It is easiest to do while in a stationary stretch position.

Begin by focusing inward and become aware of exactly where you feel the stretch.
Bring all of your attention to one spot that is tight or congested.
Stay there and gently breathe into that area—deep and slow.
Become aware of exactly how that area is feeling. Does it feel tight or clogged?
Do you feel any knots or kinks?
Do you feel any other type of discomfort?
As you inhale, imagine your breath gently sweeping through that congestion.
As your breath streams through this clogged area, visualize it dissolving the congestion.
Then as you exhale, visualize your breath carrying out the toxins from that area.

Once you breathe into it several times and feel a release, use your breath to let go further into the stretch.

The object is to give complete focus to one area at a time and nourish and cleanse it with your breath. This takes a good amount of concentration. Be patient, and don't expect results right away. It can take days, months, or years to clear congestion. Just remember, the benefits are cumulative, so perseverance and patience are necessary.

SEVEN *heart activation*

"It is only with the heart that one can see rightly;

what is essential is invisible to the eye."—ANTOINE DE SAINT-EXUPERY

Inside each one of us is an amazing energy that can turn a negative into a positive or a bad day into a good one. It can transform our state of being and put us into alignment with our inner strength and power. This beautiful energy lies within our heart space and is often referred to as our heart energy or heart intelligence. It's a high-speed intuitive source of wisdom and clear perception, an intelligence that embraces and fosters both mental and emotional intelligence.[1] When our mental and emotional intelligence comes into alignment we dance through life with a sense of faith and buoyancy. Everything falls into place because we are internally coherent and when a system is coherent all of its components are operating in harmony.

In Essential Stretch the heart is seen as the intuitive director. Through movement and internal focus we tap into our natural sense of feeling. This helps us connect with our body and heart. Once we are tapped in it is easier to be guided in the right direction, through our stretches as well as through life. There has been a lot of scientific research done on this subject, indicating that the heart is an intuitive source guiding us to the right choices. If you're interested in more scientific detail regarding the heart, I suggest you pick up a book called *The HeartMath Solution*.

For centuries many ancient cultures, poets, and philosophers have regarded the heart as the center of our lives. The Mesopotamians, the Egyptians, the Babylonians, and the Greeks all believed the heart was capable of influencing and directing emotions, morality, and decision-making ability. In the Kabbalah the heart is considered to hold the key to the mysteries of radiant health, joy, and well-being. In Chinese medicine the heart is seen as the seat of connection between the mind and the body, forming a bridge between the two. Yogis believe that the heart is what guides us to attainment of bodily equilibrium and balance. They see the heart as the seat of individual consciousness.

Modern day scientists are now validating what many of the ancient philosophers knew. Neuroscientists have discovered that the heart has its own independent nervous system referred to as "the brain in the heart." There are at least forty thousand neurons (nerve cells) in the heart—as many as are found in various subcortical centers in the brain.[2]

Most of us are driven from our thinking minds, rather than our intuitive hearts. The part of our mind that wants the control is sometimes referred to as our ego or our false self. The challenge is to recognize when our ego is trying to run the show and then be able to shift to our heart. If we could just let our heart sit in the driver's seat and guide our thinking mind in the right direction, we would experience more clarity and harmony, as our heart is connected to the divine order of the universe.

Becoming more awake to the power of your heart is a process that requires attention. If you want to develop greater intuition and learn to decipher truth from illusion, practicing heart activation can point you in the right direction. To activate our heart energy we first must learn to focus our attention on our heart alone.

In the process of Essential Stretch we are training ourselves to connect to our heart. Each time we mindfully stretch we take ourselves out of our head and into our body and heart, which can happen effortlessly because of the relaxing nature of the oscillations.

As we relax we are better able to open up to our heart and access this beautiful source of energy; as we align ourselves with our heart energy we can experience greater healing. The heart sees beyond the illusions of human drama and the ego, raising us above the rubbish that blocks our blessings. As we sharpen this connection to our heart we open up for greater intuition and positive guidance. Optimally our heart and our brain work as a team. Shifting focus from the head to the heart improves nervous system balance, heightens cardiovascular efficiency, and enhances communication between the heart and brain, bringing more coherence to the mind and emotions.[3]

Tapping into your heart becomes easier with practice. Simply putting your intention and energy toward your heart is a good beginning. Your heart is powerful, intelligent, loving, and compassionate. Merely recognizing and bringing your attention to it will begin to ignite the light of intuitive wisdom. With persistence and consistency, your heart will guide you from a place of intuitive knowledge that is in sync with the divine order of the universe. Ultimately you want to be tapped into your heart as much as possible. Stretch and meditation give you time to nurture that connection and practice tapping in. Be patient, and tap in often for best results. Try the following techniques one at a time.

Heart Hug

Most people find this the easiest way to tap into their heart, so this is a good one to start with. You can do this standing, sitting, or lying down.

1   Wrap your arms around yourself at the level of your heart.

2   Close your eyes and focus into your heart. Feel as though you're loving, nurturing, and embracing your heart.

3   With each breath allow yourself to sink deeper into your heart space.

4   Recall a situation when you felt extremely appreciative, happy, or loving.

5   Notice how that feels in your heart. Stay there as long as you need to really connect with that feeling.

6   Let go of the circumstance you envisioned and continue to experience that feeling of love, joy, or appreciation in your heart.

7 Remember these qualities are in your heart always. The exterior circumstance and your attention just activated what is already within you. You can activate this yourself anytime.

HEALING PARTS OF YOUR BODY THROUGH HEART ACTIVATION:

Single Position Stretch

This can be done in any stretch position.

1 Go into a stretch position.

2 Observe your body and notice any areas of tightness or tension.

3 Bring your mind into a specific area that you would like to work on.

4 Pay attention to what it feels like in that area.

5 Now bring your focus into your heart.

6 Once you feel tapped into your heart begin to visualize with your breath: Inhale into your heart and as you exhale, send your heart energy into that area of your body you are working on.

7 Repeat this process as many times as you would like. Notice how your body feels through each repetition.

Oscillations

It is a bit more difficult to do heart activation during oscillations only because there is more to do in each moment. During a heart-activated oscillation you are weaving together your mind, body, breath, heart, and movement. I would suggest trying this after you are very familiar with the choreography, so you don't have to think about the movement.

1 Do your first oscillation. Using your breath and observing your body through the movement, notice any areas that seem blocked or congested.

2 The second time you go through your oscillation, in conjunction with the movement inhale into your heart and exhale your heart energy into those areas of congestion.

3   Repeat this process as many times as you would like. Notice how your body feels through each repetition. Does it get easier? Do you feel a release?

The Inner Smile

The inner smile is a symbol that can assist in activating your heart energy. This is a very gentle way of connecting the mind and body and bringing joy into a specific area of the body. The energy of joy is healing and is something that we already have within us in our hearts—we just have to activate it. Through visualization we consciously prepare ourselves so that eventually it blends with what we already have within. One of my favorite meditation teachers, Karl Schleinig, introduced me to this method. He uses the inner smile to help open the chakras, the body's energy centers. Many Taoist masters use this technique to heal different organs in the body. We use it in Essential Stretch to relax the muscles and assist in opening areas of stuck energy.

I   Once you are in your stretch position, focus into your body.

2   Notice any tightness or discomfort in your body.

3   Take a moment to focus your attention wherever you felt the discomfort.

4   Inhale focusing into your heart space.

5   Gently send a smile into that area where you felt the tightness. It can be your smile or someone else's smile or a smile you create.

EIGHT *meditation*

"Meditation has to do with opening what is closed in us, balancing what is reactive, and exploring and investigating what is hidden. That is the why of practice. We practice to open, to balance and to explore."—JACK KORNFIELD

Meditation allows the mind to rest, relax, and rejuvenate. It's a process of letting go of thoughts concerning the exterior and focusing inward. It allows our mind to take a break from surface mind-chatter. During this break we open the channels to our heaven within, tapping in to our true self, our true essence. This is our power center, our inner strength, our infinite wisdom, and our natural creativity. This is a beautiful space from which to live.

The power or energy that creates everything in nature is the same energy that lies within each one of us. Tapping into this source unites us with all things and aligns us with the universe. In the surrender of our human control we ascend the stairway to universal harmony and get the answers for which we've been yearning. As the bible says, "Be still and know."

But if the answers are within us, why is it so hard to grasp them? Why is life so confusing at times? The busyness of our minds can be like clutter in a closet. In a huge mess we have trouble finding something that is right in front of us; similarly, the clutter in our minds can block the natural flow of life. When we are relaxed and open, we fall into alignment with all things and life seems to unfold effortlessly. Opportunities come to us. We don't have to chase down and control everything. There is a divine order in this universe and we are more able to participate in that as we open ourselves up to it.

So how do we open up? How do we become clear? How can we live in this great field of infinite possibilities, or as Deepak Chopra calls it, "the field of infinite potentiality"? There are many different methods of cleansing the mind and body and I suggest you try a variety of methods from sound healing to nutritional cleansing, as every little bit helps. For the purpose of this book we'll stick with stretch. Both stretching and meditation are cleansing and help to open us up, and when we combine the two the rewards are even greater!

incorporating meditation while stretching

Essential Stretch is a movement meditation. The technique is grounded in mind/body connection. Practicing it on a regular basis will have just as great an effect on your mind as it does on your body. The practice will help you learn how to drop all thought and focus on each moment. You will learn how to use your breath as the thread connecting your mind to your body and your body to the energy current of the movement. Before you know it, your mind, body, breath, and movement will be woven together into effortless movement meditation. Essential Stretch also eliminates blockages, toxins, and negative energy. This release opens doorways into our true self. By peeling back the layers of human drama, Essential Stretch takes you closer to your inner self and therefore everything else in this universe.

While you stretch:

Let go of all exterior distractions, thought, and mind-chatter, and bring all your attention into your body.

Follow and feel every little part of the movement.
Stay present in each moment of the stretch.

As you focus in your body, you open those areas up to be bathed with attention and healing energy. Connecting your mind and body allows you to halt mind-chatter and nurture specific areas of the body.

POST STRETCH MEDITATION

Taking time to meditate at the end of your stretch workout can be very beneficial. Since your mind and body are more relaxed when you finish stretching, you'll find it easier to be still. If you have never meditated before, start with about five minutes, and as you feel ready slowly increase your time. The more often you meditate, the easier it will be to let go of surface mind-chatter, although every day will be different. Some days you'll feel as though you're wrestling your thoughts to no avail. Don't worry—don't get discouraged and don't judge yourself. The fact that you are putting time into meditation is enough to reap benefits.

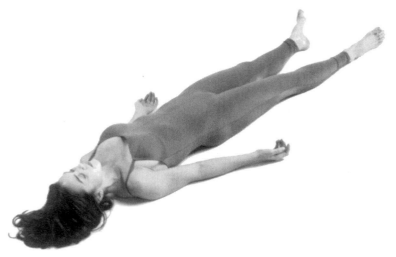

You can meditate sitting or lying down, but either way try to stay alert. If you find yourself zoning out or falling asleep while lying down, you may want to try sitting. Or you may need to rest. Take a nap and meditate after. It is best to be in a position where your spine is straight. If sitting unsupported bothers your back try sitting against a wall or in a chair with a straight back.

There are several ways to assist the emptying or quieting of your mind in meditation. Here are a few methods for you to try.

1   Focus on your breathing and allow your breath to carry you inward. Don't try to control your breathing, simply observe it. When you're meditating you're not trying to do anything, you are completely surrendering. Just be.

2   Repeat a mantra in your head, such as "I am," or "one, two." Pointing your mind to one thing often helps quiet the chatter. Once the mantra has stilled your mind, you can let go of the mantra and just be.

3   Ask to be empty. Then if your mind begins to wander and thoughts start entering simply observe them, but don't entertain the thoughts. Don't do anything with the thoughts because then you are giving them power. Simply be the observer without feeding it and without judging it.

Following meditation, we often feel more peaceful and move from that sacred space within us. As we move from that space within we are able to see more clearly and be more open for divine direction. This allows us to make decisions from a space of clarity not chaos, to flow from a space of unlimited wisdom and creativity, to come from love not fear. With consistent meditation practice we align ourselves with our true essence and all things in the universe, our vision of all possibilities expands and we are unrestricted by our egos. To further facilitate openness to all possibilities, you may want to write down your discoveries in a journal. By disclosing the treasures of your innermost self onto paper you create a visual imprint on the mind, thereby helping you manifest the dreams of your heart into your life. Allow your thoughts to flow freely onto the pages, completely unrestricted. This is key in personal growth.

Your endless resources,
Are deeper than the sea,
And they flow like a river,
When you let go and just be.

NINE *centering*

"Know thyself and thou shalt know the universe."—SOCRATES

Centering is the ability to direct your mental focus from the outer world to your inner world. As you will discover, stretching itself will help to center you, but if you take a few moments to center yourself before you dive into your workout your rewards will multiply tremendously. Ideally you want to let go of all exterior distractions so you can reach that quiet, centered place inside. "Exterior distractions" might include noise, someone in the next room, a radio playing in the background, or anything going on in your own mind.

For instance, if you have a busy, chaotic, or even frustrating day, your inner dialogue could be busy judging or discussing the events of the day—maybe without your conscious awareness. When you stop to center yourself, notice your mind. What's going on up there? Is it busy chattering away about the day? Are there some worries about the future floating around in your mind? All of this mind-chatter creates confusion and gets in the way of our focus and concentration.

Centering before you stretch gives you a moment to remind yourself that the chaos of the day does not belong in this space. If you must, you can pick it back up after your workout. As you are able to move away from the busyness of the day, it becomes easier to relax and move into your heart and your body. A relaxed state is conducive to clearer focus and deeper stretching. Optimally, through centering you will train yourself to move into a calm and receptive state and get the most out of your stretch.

Stretching also provides a great opportunity to work on transforming your thoughts from negative, or self-sabotaging, to positive, or constructive contemplation. By using the tools explained below you can increase your self-awareness and set specific goals to catapult your growth. Through stretching you become more in touch with yourself and more aware of what needs work. As you clear your consciousness and transform binding thoughts into open optimism, life becomes more harmonious, peaceful, and joyful. This doesn't happen overnight—be patient. Over time and with consistency, centering yourself will increase your ability to connect and transform. To do this properly, you'll need to be honest with yourself and take responsibility for your own consciousness. If you see your thoughts are on the greedy or jealous side, admit it to yourself and use that self-knowledge in your intention to transform. It's not always easy taking a look at ourselves because we don't want to see our dark side. But if we choose to take responsibility, we can transform the darkness to light. The tools below are designed to help you on your unique path, but ultimately it is up to you. You are the only one who can transform your life.

This centering technique includes four parts, which you can carry throughout your life to guide you in the right direction. As you become more proficient through practice, they will flow simultaneously.

1   Increase your self-awareness

2   Quiet your mind

3   Focus inward

4   Create a positive shift

ONE: *Increase your self-awareness*

This is a critical part of the process. If you are oblivious of your mind's activity you can't create a positive shift simply because you don't know what you have to shift. Observing your mind will tell you a lot about yourself; your thoughts are the invisible blueprint of your life. Whatever is occupying your mind the most is what you bring into your life either directly or indirectly. For example, if you spend your time thinking about how you lack the skills for a particular job or how your limited knowledge will prevent you from getting a promotion, the qualities of lack and limitation will resonate in your work. Self-observation is step one in cleaning up mind-rubbish. It is only when you know what needs to be cleaned up that you can begin to work toward a clear mind.

To observe your thoughts, take yourself out of your mind's conversation and become a witness to the activity. Notice the dialogue and how you entertain your thoughts. For instance, if this thought were to come into your mind, "I'm never going to have enough time to complete my tasks today," notice what your mind does from there. Does it begin to entertain that thought by going through all the tasks you need to do? Do you become overwhelmed by the mere thoughts of your workload? Thoughts can be counterproductive, taking you out of the moment, possibly creating anxiety and robbing your mind, body, and soul of energy.

TWO: *Quiet your mind*

The object here is to let go of your ego, that part of you that doubts and offers resistance. For some of you, once you see how unnecessary these thoughts are, you may find it easy to drop the chatter or stop entertaining them. For most though, it's not that simple. As you will see when you begin to work on this, it's difficult to empty the mind. But when you do, you let go of control and open the space to be in alignment with universal harmony. You create the space to receive. In Zen, this is called the "don't know mind." Zen masters have long taught the benefits of approaching life with an empty mind to be more receptive and open for the seeds of opportunity.

THREE: Focus inward

The object is to focus inward and connect to your heart space. As you train your mind to concentrate on your heart, you take yourself out of your head and therefore quiet the mind.

FOUR: Create a positive shift

This step allows you to set an intention regarding what you want to achieve during your workout. In this step you create a positive shift in your consciousness. You take your challenges and counter them with a positive statement designed to help you rise above your current situation: if your current situation is lack, you focus on abundance, if it's confusion, you focus on clarity. Basically we're trying to rise above all the muck in our minds by bringing our attention to a quality that is the positive opposite. You may be comfortable with creating your own centering statements; however, if the statements or prayers below resonate with you, use them. Each statement below has a different purpose. Choose whatever area you want to work on that day or substitute your own words into one of the following to customize your own centering statement.

Begin by closing your eyes and focusing into your heart space.

Breathe into your heart a few times until you feel connected.

Say your prayer with conviction, knowing that this is what you intend to do in this stretch session.

When you are finished with your centering statement, take another deep breath into your heart and solidify your intention.

Then begin your stretch workout.

CLARITY

Take this moment to simply let go of any worldly distractions and focus inward, recognizing the beautiful space that lies within me. I know that beyond the fogginess of my mind there is clarity, there is focus, and there is infinite intelligence. I know that through this workout any stress, any anxiety, anything weighing heavily on my mind or body will simply melt away with the movement. I am clearing my body and quieting my mind, rediscovering my natural state of being, so that I may live from clarity, not chaos. For this and so much more, I am grateful . . . and I allow it to be.

LETTING GO OF BURDENS

As I take this time to let go of any burdens I'm carrying, I realize they are either baggage from the past or worries concerning the future. Both rob my mind and body of energy and vitality, and weigh heavily on my life, so through this workout I release and let go of this heaviness as I focus on the moment. As I lay down my burdens I become lighter, feeling and sensing the beautiful buoyancy of the moment and cherishing it—just the way it is. In gratitude and thanksgiving, I release my burdens . . . knowing it is already done.

SELF-LOVE

I simply take this time for myself to focus into my heart space. For I know that all of the love, peace, joy, and beauty that I need is right here, right now—within me. I let go of any self-judgment, knowing that judgment alone blocks my ability to shine from my heart space. And as I massage my body with movement, I unblock anything that is obstructing my highest good. For this and so much more I am grateful and I simply allow it to be.

PEACE

I simply take this moment to turn within, feeling, sensing, and accepting the calm nature of my spirit, knowing that the stress and chaos that appears on the outside of my life is not who I am on the inside. I allow this workout to clear the clutter out of my mind and body so that I may come from a space of peace. For this and so much more I am eternally grateful and I simply allow it to be.

MIND/BODY CONNECTION

As I take this moment to quiet my mind and focus inward, I become keenly aware of my breath, knowing that through each stretch I allow my breath to be the thread that connects my mind to my body, recognizing that in this workout and through my life, my mind and body work as a team. I give thanks for this beautiful, harmonious partnership, knowing that this work results in perfect balance, peace, and harmony. In complete gratitude I simply allow it to be.

BEING HAPPY

I simply take this time to recognize the beautiful spirit that I am. I know that as I continue to tap into my body and my heart during this stretch I strengthen my connection to my inner self and increase my ability to allow my spirit to shine through me as I dance through life in bliss. The more open I become, the brighter I allow my spirit to shine through and sprinkle happiness upon my life and the lives of others. For this and so much more I am grateful and I simply allow it to be.

SHORT CENTERING STATEMENTS

I give thanks for this time that I'm giving myself to open up and become more in touch with my inner guidance.

I am so very grateful to have this time to nurture my mind/body/spirit connection so that I can feed my whole person.

Through this stretch workout that I am about to experience, I let go of all the rubbish in my mind so that I can float through life freely.

I simply take this time to shed the stress and anxiety that is weighing me down, so that I can feel buoyant and joyful.

I am so very grateful to have this time to relax my mind and body and open up to the natural flow of my creativity.

PART FOUR

the stretches

"The healthy body is a flowing, interactive electrodynamic energy field. Motion is more natural to life than non-motion—things that keep flowing are inherently good. What interferes with flow will have detrimental effects."—VALERIE V. HUNT

Approach your stretch program with an open and kind mind. Accept exactly where you are and become keenly aware of that by noticing your body through each stretch. Everyone's body is different. You could be really flexible in one area, and super tight in another area. So as you begin to try different stretches be gentle with yourself. Be aware of how your body feels through the movement and never force a stretch; the Tao of the movement is enough to flush congestion and open you up. In fact, you will receive greater rewards if you approach Essential Stretching in a relaxed and gentle manner. Look for progress, not perfection.

Be easy on yourself upstairs too—don't judge yourself. It's not about how flexible you are. It's most important to sharpen your mind/body connection and nurture your-self through regular stretching. This does not mean rush through a stretch at the end of your workout. If you really want to relieve stress, restore vibrant health, sharpen mental alertness, and achieve many of the other amazing stretch benefits, you've got to make it a lifestyle. Listen to your body, take it one step at a time, and enjoy the process of freeing yourself through movement!

DO I NEED TO WARM UP BEFORE I STRETCH?

It is more effective to stretch warm muscles; however, oscillations with a large range of motion help to generate the flow of qi throughout your body, which helps to warm you up. Your muscles are more pliable when they are warm and therefore will expand more easily. Be aware of where you are starting (the state of your body) and what your purpose is. If you've just come inside from a cold winter day and you're looking to increase flexibility, it's advantageous to take at least five minutes to walk, dance, jog in place, or any other movement that warms your body. Then you can allow the oscillations to take over and continue to raise the core temperature of the body.

You may notice as your body gets clearer that you require less of a warm-up. Though warming up will still facilitate a deeper stretch, regular stretching promotes healthy and supple muscles and allows for greater freedom of movement even when you haven't warmed up. With consistency, you will find the stretches getting easier.

If you're just taking a quick stretch break you can do most oscillations without warming up, but remember to be very gentle on your body. Quick stretches are mainly designed to relieve stress and prevent stagnation and keep the body open for the flow of qi, though the accumulation of lots of short stretch breaks throughout the day will add to your flexibility.

Anytime you're working with this type of movement with an inward focus, based on feeling and sensitivity, you connect to various psychophysical parts of yourself and different emotions may arise. At times you may feel like giggling, and other times you may feel like crying. I encourage you to allow yourself to feel these emotions without judgment. Let yourself just be with the process. Emotions come up to heal and pass, so it's not advisable to push them back down. Give yourself permission to express those feelings, remaining compassionate and loving throughout your process. The movement in the oscillations will help to move this emotional energy out, so take your time and stay in the moment.

> "Michelle's powerful stretch technique transforms at every level.
> As I see where I am holding or gripping in my body,
> I learn how I am holding and gripping in my life.
> By stretching and sending energy to those places
> I open in the same way a flower blossoms."
> —MERE LATOUR

Tips and Reminders:

- Always try to be present or mindful while stretching.

- Muscles that are warm are more pliable and easier to stretch.

- It helps to center yourself before stretching.

- Listen to your body and give yourself extra time on tighter areas.

- Always do what "feels" right. If it's painful, don't do it. Modify the stretch or opt for another exercise.

- Stay free of judgments regarding your body and your flexibility in order to remain open for healing.

- Focus on the area you are stretching, feeling and sensing each part of the stretch. Is it tense or gripping or is it relaxed and open for the stretch? Make any necessary adjustments to relax the muscles you're stretching.

- Notice the rest of your body. How is it feeling? Is it tight or constricted in any way? If so, make any necessary adjustments to take pressure off those areas.

- Pay close attention to the process and quality of your movement.

- Once you are comfortable with the stretches, try closing your eyes. This not only helps you focus inward, but also heightens your mind/body awareness through feeling and sensing.

- You increase your stretch effectiveness when you open the pathway from the crown to the root (along the spine) in the beginning of your workout. (Examples: Spinal Roll, Standing Caterpillar.)

- Try to slow down and deepen your breathing as you progress through your stretch workout.

TEN *full body stretches*

The oscillations in this chapter take you through a range of motion that stretches many muscles in the body. Use the illustrations as a guideline for the pattern of movement and work through your own personal range of motion (PROM). You do not have to achieve the same range of motion shown in this book to get results. Measure your range by feel and simply go to the point of mild discomfort—not pain!

Whether you're doing an oscillation in a seated, standing, or lying down position, one of the biggest challenges is to relax your body. Observe your body through each oscillation, noticing any areas where you may be holding or gripping muscles and try to consciously relax those areas. Generally the only muscles you will need to contract while stretching are your abdominal muscles in order to keep your center of balance.

Spinal roll

NECK, BACK, GLUTES, AND HAMSTRINGS

BENEFITS This movement tops the list for something you can do anytime throughout the day to release tension and rejuvenate. By loosening the muscles in the neck and back, you can relieve tension and anxiety that commonly nests in those areas and restricts natural movement, robs the body of energy, and blocks proper functioning of the nervous system. The Spinal Roll clears congested tension, augmenting your freedom of movement, coordination, agility, and flexibility.

Communication systems along the spine conduct messages to the rest of the body. When the spine is obstructed with anxiety, tension, and tightness, messages do not flow through as freely and efficiently and you may not feel as sharp and quick. These blockages impede our mind/body communication and slow down everything we do, including functions of which we are not consciously aware, such as circulation and the transfer of nourishment to organs. The Spinal Roll stimulates the flow of energy and fluids through the spine, nourishing and rejuvenating spinal nerves and awakening systems in the spine that transmit messages to the rest of the body.

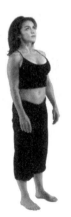 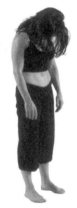 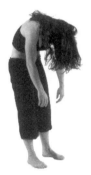 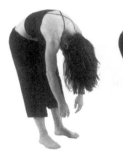

1. Stand straight with your feet shoulder distance apart.

2. Gently bring your chin to your chest.

- Relax the muscles in the back of your neck.

3. Let your shoulders collapse forward.

- Relax the muscles in your upper back, shoulders, and arms.

4. Allow your knees to bend gradually as you continue to round forward.

- Relax all the muscles through your back.

- Roll back up in the same slow fashion.

"My spine is alive, healthy, and whole and a beautiful conductor of messages to the rest of my body."

Diagonal Spinal Roll

NECK, BACK, GLUTES, AND HAMSTRINGS

BENEFITS This stretch can be considered a variation of the Spinal Roll. While you still receive all of the beautiful benefits of the Spinal Roll, the Diagonal Roll adds an additional range of motion, expanding the stretch farther out from the spine on each side. This is particularly helpful for those who tend to be tight in the rhomboids and lower back area.

This stretch is most effective when performed in conjunction with the Spinal Roll. As a pair they can be done anytime for instant relief of stiffness and stress.

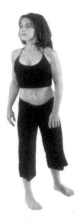 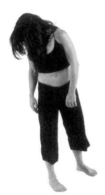 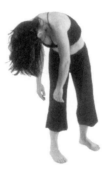 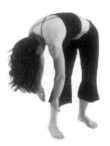 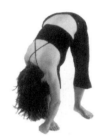

1. Stand straight with your feet shoulder distance apart, and turn your shoulders and hips to face diagonal right.

2. Bring your chin to your chest.
- Let go of the muscles in the back of your neck.

3. Allow your shoulders to collapse forward.
- Let go through your upper back, shoulders, and arms.

4. Continue to roll down through the center of your back.
- Allow your knees to bend and arms to hang loosely while you relax your entire back.

5. Roll down into your lower back.
- Increase the bend in your knees if you need to.
- Slowly roll up in the same loose fashion.
- Repeat to the left.

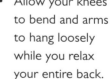

"I am so very grateful to be nurturing my body right now."

Standing Caterpillar

NECK, BACK, GLUTES, AND HAMSTRINGS

BENEFITS This stretch feeds the spine with both activation and relaxation. The first part of this movement, flat back forward, subtly activates the muscles through the back as you carry your body forward. This warms and nourishes the spinal nerves, muscles, and ligaments by circulating blood into that area. When the erector spinae (the muscles next to the spine) are contracted for a few seconds it actually makes it easier to relax those muscles in the next phase of the stretch where you let go in your neck, shoulders, arms, and back. As you roll up loosely, fluids and energy are flushed through the back, cleansing and opening lines of communication throughout the mental, physical, and emotional body.

This exercise does a wonderful job educating the back muscles to keep the spine aligned properly while increasing elasticity. The Standing Caterpillar can be done anytime and is extremely beneficial when performed on a daily basis.

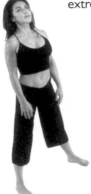

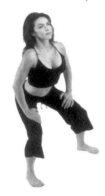

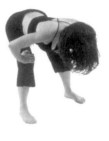

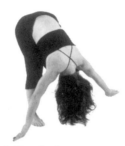

3. Lengthen forward with a flat back (or arch if it's comfortable).

4. Gently drop your arms and head toward the ground.

1. Stand tall with feet shoulders distance apart.

2. Bend your knees, allowing your hands to slide down your thighs for support.

"I let go of all self-judgment and allow myself to enjoy my body through movement."

6. Finish in your starting position.

- Breathe deeply throughout the entire movement.

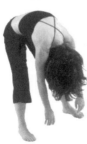

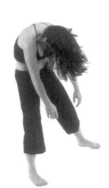

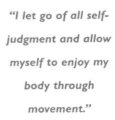

5. Roll up one vertebra at a time.

Single Leg Caterpillar

HAMSTRINGS, BACK, NECK, CALVES, AND GLUTES

BENEFITS This convenient oscillation can be done anywhere and anytime. You don't have to get down on the floor, and you don't have to warm up prior to executing this one. Do this at the office, on a plane, or even in a store. You can go as deep or shallow as you'd like with this stretch. This is a great stretch to use in your warm-up for almost all sports and activities.

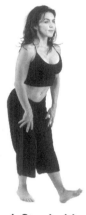

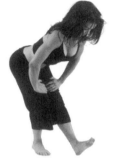

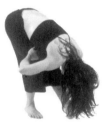

1. Stand with your knees bent and extend your left leg, placing your heel on the ground in front of you.

- Your extended leg is straight with a soft knee (do not lock the knee) and a flexed foot.

2. Lengthen forward and place your hands on your thighs for support. Keep your neck in line with your spine.

- If you need to, allow your extended knee to bend.

- Lengthen your body down toward your leg.

3. Once you are at your maximum stretch, drop your head.

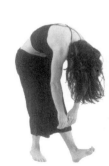

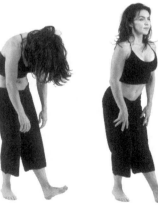

4. Roll up gradually, one vertebra at a time.

5. Bring your head up last.
- Repeat to the right side.

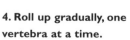

"I no longer waste my time, energy, and creative mind on worries."

Side Sway

TORSO, LATS, WAIST, AND SHOULDERS

BENEFITS You may get a little surprise when you try this one for your first time. It looks simple, yet most people have quite a lack of mobility down the side of their body. Since this exercise involves most of the torso and moves from one side to another, it benefits everything from the shoulders down to the hips and from the abs to the back. It not only stretches, but also sculpts and tones the waist and abdominals.

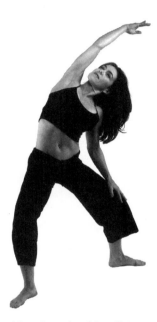

Stand with your legs slightly wider than shoulder distance apart. Feet can be turned out or forward, whatever is comfortable for you. Bend both knees and feel yourself rooted into the ground. Reach your right arm over your head and as far as you can toward the left side.

- Use your left hand on your thigh for support.

- Allow your arms to gracefully open as you repeat to the other side.

"I treat my body with care and respect, knowing it is a divine instrument for my spirit to shine through."

Multi-level Circles *(Levels: Neck, Upper Back, Mid Back, Lower Back)*

NECK, ENTIRE TORSO AND BACK INCLUDING: TRAPS, RHOMBOIDS, ERECTOR SPINAE, LATS, REAR DELTS, WAIST, GLUTES, AND HAMSTRINGS

BENEFITS A great opener for all the muscles in the torso! Do this in the beginning and end of any workout (after the Spinal and Diagonal Spinal Rolls). Large circular movements increase qi and blood flow, warming, cleansing, and nourishing the entire body. Since this stretch covers the whole torso, it enhances freedom of movement for dancing, martial arts, basketball, tennis, and any other activities that can improve with greater range of motion.

This oscillation can also prevent neck and back kinks or spasms, which seem to pop up out of nowhere. The reality of this common kink is it usually brews from stress upon stress. Without any form of release, such as stretching, the knot gets worse and finally spasms, leaving a person in extreme pain and unable to turn his or her head. Sound familiar? Everyone has had a stiff neck at least once or twice—stretching regularly can help prevent that.

This oscillation does a great job readjusting and balancing the body. The movement is like a pendulum and, with repetition, equalizes and harmonizes the entire system.

NOTE: **Before performing this oscillation, do the Spinal Roll and Diagonal Spinal Roll to prepare your neck and back for this deeper stretch. This is also not an easy stretch. Take your time and don't go beyond your personal range of motion.**

- Throughout this movement, the direction of your body and face remains front.
- All of your joints should be soft.
- Let go of the muscles in your neck.
- Let your arms hang loosely.
- I include only four stages in this oscillation, but if you'd like to go deeper and add stages in between—go for it!

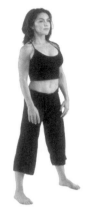

1. Begin by standing with your feet slightly wider than shoulder distance.

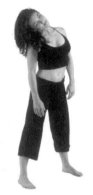

2. Gently bring your right ear to your right shoulder.

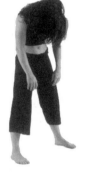

3. Gradually roll your head to the front.

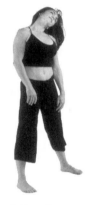

4. Continue to roll to the left side.

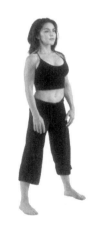

5. And then back to your neutral position.

- Do not roll your head back—only side, center, side.

- Repeat this sequence in the opposite direction.

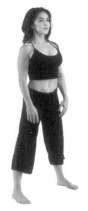

1. Begin by standing with your feet slightly wider than shoulder distance.

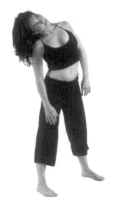

2. Gently bring your right ear to your right shoulder.

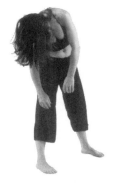

3. Roll diagonal, allowing your shoulders to collapse forward.

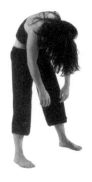

4. Continue to roll through the center and to the other side.

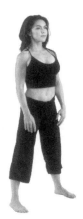

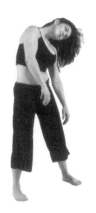

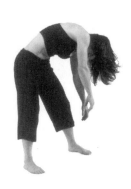

5. Return back to an upright position.

• Repeat to the other side.

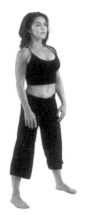

1. Begin by standing with your feet slightly wider than shoulder distance.

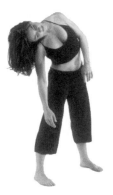

2. Bring your right ear to your right shoulder.

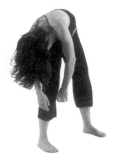

3. Allow your entire upper back to release to the diagonal.

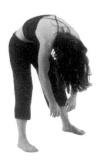

4. Then let go through the center

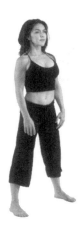

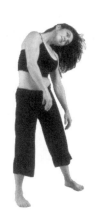

5. Continue to roll to the other side.

6. Return to your upright position.

• Repeat to the other side.

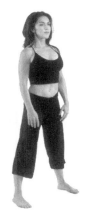

1. Begin by standing with your feet slightly wider than shoulder distance.

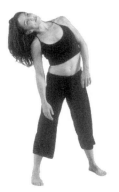

2. Bring your right ear to your right shoulder.

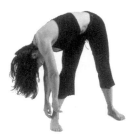

3. Allow your entire back to surrender to the diagonal.

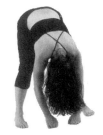

4. Smoothly move through the center.

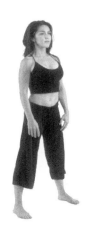

7. Finish in your upright position.

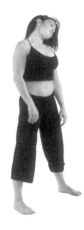

6. Rise back up on the diagonal.

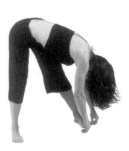

5. Continue to the other side.

"I willingly get rid of my past and stop thinking about the future, so that I can fully enjoy this moment."

Triangle

HIPS, WAIST, LATS, SHOULDERS, HAMSTRINGS, INNER THIGHS, AND LOWER BACK.

BENEFITS This is an excellent oscillation for balance, strength, and flexibility. It tones the waist, abdominals, and spinal nerves while stretching the hips, waist, lats, shoulders, hamstrings, inner thighs, and lower back. In yoga the Triangle is used to help the body become lighter and improve other asanas, which are postures, positions to be held. The object is to move through the positions effortlessly, opening the body through the movement and breath. This sequence also helps the proper functioning of the digestive system.

NOTE: Before performing this oscillation a warm-up is suggested.

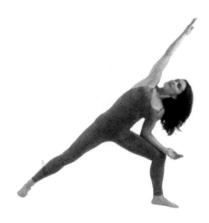

MODIFIED POSITION Use this position through the movement series if your flexibility does not allow you to open your hips and shoulders to the front with a straight leg.

- Open your legs to a comfortable wide stance.
- Turn your left foot directly out to face the side.
- Square your hips and shoulders to the front.
- Bend your left knee to no more than a 90-degree angle.
- Place your forearm on your left leg.
- Extend your right arm up to the sky, or alongside your ear if you can.

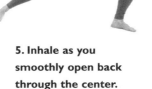

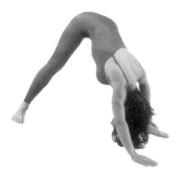

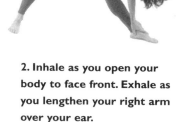

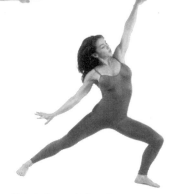

MOVEMENT SERIES

1. Begin with your feet in a comfortable wide stance, right foot facing front and left foot facing side, with your body bent forward at the hips and extended diagonal left. Your left hand is on your ankle or on the ground in front of your foot and your right hand is extended to the diagonal on the ground.

- Allow your head to drop through your shoulders.

- Let go of the muscles in the back of your neck.

2. Inhale as you open your body to face front. Exhale as you lengthen your right arm over your ear.

- Lengthen from your hips through your fingertips.

3. Inhale and simultaneously bend your left knee and travel through the center.

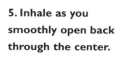

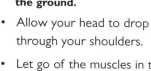

4. Exhale as you reach to the right side.

- Lengthen your waist as you reach up and over.

5. Inhale as you smoothly open back through the center.

6. Exhale as you straighten your leg and lengthen your right arm over your ear. Inhale as you roll forward toward the diagonal.

7. Exhale as you relax back into your starting position. Repeat on the other side.

"I open to reveal the true love, peace, and joy that lies within me."

full body stretches **79**

Seated Forward Bend

NECK, BACK, HAMSTRINGS, AND CALVES

BENEFITS This stretches the entire back of the body from your head to your heels and generates a considerable amount of energy flow. It invigorates the internal organs and stimulates the entire nervous system. The side-to-side rocking is a very powerful tool to further open up the lower back, hips, and glutes. When you rock, allow yourself to be loose and free and go as far as you can comfortably.

FORWARD BEND

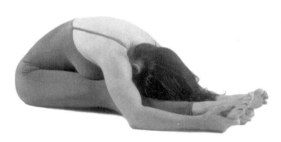

Begin sitting with your legs extended straight in front of you and relax your body forward.

- Allow your knees, ankles, and feet to be soft.
- Breathe deep and slow, allowing your lower back to expand with each breath.
- Rest in this position.

ROCKING FORWARD BEND

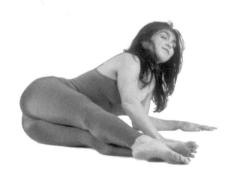

Place your hands and elbows on the ground beside your legs for support. Rock your body side to side (left and right).

- Let your leg and cheek come all the way off the ground.
- Be free—let your inner child come out!

"I let go of all surface mind-chatter, as I focus from the top of my spine all the way down to my heels."

Bird of Paradise

SHOULDERS, WAIST, BACK, GLUTES, HIPS, HAMSTRINGS, AND INNER THIGHS

BENEFITS Since this oscillation offers a new range of motion it may feel a bit awkward at first, but the benefits tremendously outweigh the initial discomfort. The sway helps bring the mind, body, and breath into one rhythm and increases energy flow, preparing the body for the roll. The roll lubricates and opens the hip and shoulder joints while stretching the entire torso. Both the sway and the roll tone the waist and help with healthy digestion. The stable base of this position frees you from the concerns of balancing or supporting the body, allowing your attention and energy to be devoted entirely to the stretch. The unique extended range of motion in this stretch is extremely effective in those with locked-up hip joints. But consistency is key—it doesn't happen after one stretch. The inner thighs are indirectly lengthened through the movement of this stretch and, though not a deep stretch for the inner thighs, it is a simpler position for most who are super tight in the hamstrings. As the hamstrings are stretched indirectly, when you go through the movement it gently flushes energy and fluids into the hamstrings to open the way for deeper stretching later in your routine. Allow your body to enjoy this blissful stretch as you open through your entire torso.

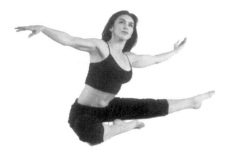 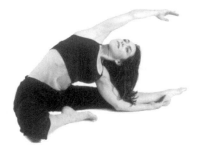

1. Begin sitting with your left leg extended straight out to the side and your right leg bent in. Your hips and shoulders are square to the front. Take a deep breath in and as you exhale, smoothly reach your right arm over your right ear toward your extended leg.

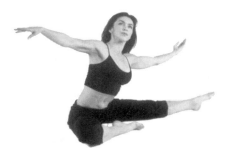 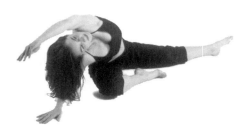

2. Inhale coming up through the center.

3. Exhale as you reach to the right.

- Continue to weave your breath through the movement, exhaling into the final stretch on each side.

- Repeat to the other side.

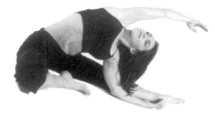

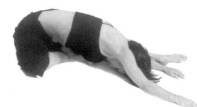

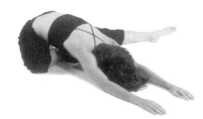

1. Exhale and extend your right arm over your right ear toward your extended leg.

2. Allow your body to slowly roll to the left diagonal.

3. Then continue the roll through the center.

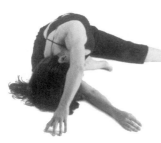

4. And to the right side to whatever point is comfortable.

- If you can, allow your left shoulder to roll up toward the sky.

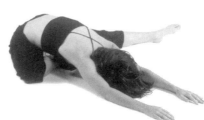

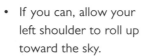

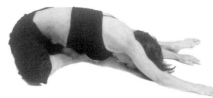

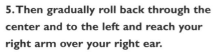

5. Then gradually roll back through the center and to the left and reach your right arm over your right ear.

- Repeat four to eight full oscillations on each side.

"I allow my body to be buoyant and free as I eliminate the stress through my stretch."

full body stretches **83**

Butterfly

NECK, BACK, INNER THIGHS, HIPS, AND GLUTES

BENEFITS The Butterfly is an excellent oscillation for mind/body breath awareness. The contraction part of the movement stimulates energy flow and stretches the back of the neck, trapezius, rhomboids, and upper to middle erector spinae (the muscles next to the spine). As you round forward, energy is pushed down the erector spinae into the lower back, hips, and glutes and then driven into the legs. Scooping up completes the circle and keeps energy flowing in a circular motion. This movement gently forces the hips to shift back and forth, assisting in opening the hips and glutes and allowing the energy to pass through into the legs. The Butterfly helps to open up, rebalance, and realign the lower back and hips, and increases sensitivity, awareness, and flexibility.

Grasping your ankles gives you leverage to increase the stretch in the upper back, spreading the scapula and deepening the stretch in the rhomboids. The rhomboids are a common home for knots and anxiety. This stretch can help to smooth out those knots and calm anxiety.

BUTTERFLY CONTRACTION

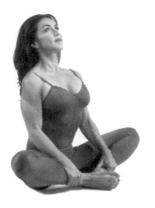 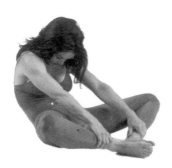 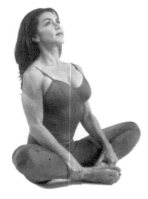

1. Sit tall with your knees open, the soles of your feet together, and your hands grasping your ankles (Butterfly position).

- Lengthen your neck and relax your shoulders back.

2. Inhale, sit up straight, and exhale and contract back (rounding your back), bringing your chin to your chest.

- Feel the stretch down through your neck and back.

3. Inhale as you sit back up into your starting position.

- Repeat several times, synchronizing your breath with the movement.

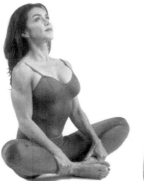

1. Sit tall in Butterfly position.

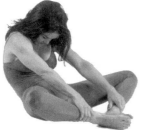

2. Inhale, sit up straight, exhale and contract back (rounding your back, chin to your chest).

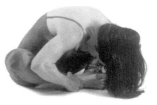

3. Gradually round forward, bringing your head toward your feet.

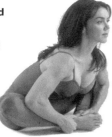

4. Scoop up starting with your head (forehead, nose, then chin)

"I cherish that which is within me."

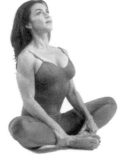

5. Allow your body to follow. Finish in your starting position.
• Repeat several times.

Clam, Open Clam, and Clam Roll

CLAM: LOWER BACK, BUTTOCKS, AND INSERTION POINT OF HAMSTRINGS

OPEN CLAM AND CLAM ROLL: NECK, BACK, AND GLUTES

BENEFITS This is a nice leisurely way to stretch your back. Lying on your back and bringing your knees in to your chest is a great position to ground and center yourself. In this position the ground provides straight support for your spine, while gravity works in your favor helping to flatten your back against the floor. Simply by bending your legs into your body, you gently massage abdominal muscles and the digestive system helping to release any excess air from the intestines. This stretch is especially wonderful to do before rising in the morning to stretch your lower back and before retiring at night to ease the day's tensions in the back and stomach.

By curling up into a basket you bring the rest of the back and neck into the stretch. Then rolling your body forward and back is an excellent movement for ironing out the kinks in your back. With the roll, you create a steady stream of light pressure as each part of your back smoothly rolls across the ground. This gently massages the spinal vertebrae, back muscles, and surrounding ligaments. This movement helps to get rid of any stiffness in the spine and stimulates the nerves running alongside.

CLAM

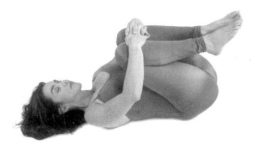

Begin lying on your back and bend your knees into your chest.

- Wrap your hands around your legs.

- Allow your back to melt down into the ground.

- Breathe.

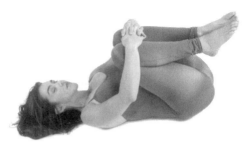

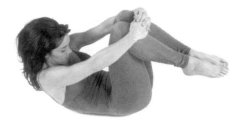

1. Begin lying on your back and bend your knees into your chest. Slowly move your knees away from your chest.

- Allow your arms to straighten and interlace your fingertips around your knees.

2. Gradually bring your chin to your chest and raise your upper back off the ground.

- Breathe from your neck down to your tailbone.
- Then slowly flatten your back to the mat.
- Repeat as much as your heart desires!

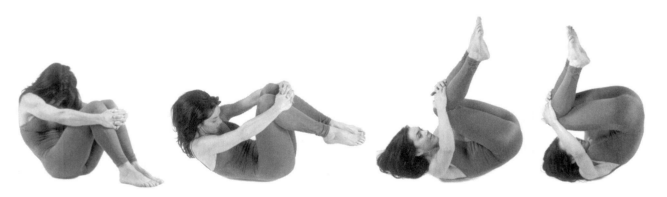

Holding on to your knees, allow your body to roll freely forward and back.

- Smooth and soothe your back through the rock!

"I have the courage to continue to walk in the direction of surrender."

full body stretches **87**

Spinal Twist

CHEST, ANTERIOR DELTS, BACK, GLUTES, AND HIPS

BENEFITS Many stretches bend the body forward and back, but to truly become flexible the spine must be twisted laterally as well. Twisting the spine actually helps to align the spine. So if you need a little adjustment, don't be surprised if you hear a little cracking along your spine as you do this stretch. It is important that you are warm when you do this, and that you don't force the stretch. If your body is open enough and ready to realign itself, it will happen naturally with the gentle twist. This also rejuvenates and tones spinal nerves and ligaments and improves digestion.

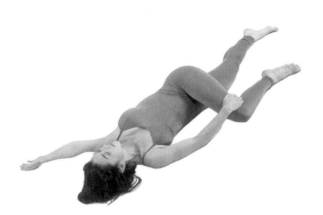

Begin lying on your back with both legs extended out straight and bring your left knee into your chest. Cross your left leg across your body.

- Extend your left arm straight out to the left.

- Allow your body to melt down into the ground.

- Calmly follow your breath down your spine.

- Repeat to the other side.

"As I align my spine, I quiet my mind and align myself with the universe."

Body Yawn *Supine extension*

FULL BODY

BENEFITS This is a great stretch to wake up and enliven your body from head to toe. It is also a great position to visualize energy flowing through your body to get your mind and body working together.

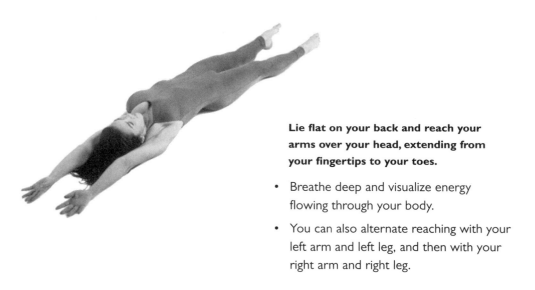

Lie flat on your back and reach your arms over your head, extending from your fingertips to your toes.

- Breathe deep and visualize energy flowing through your body.

- You can also alternate reaching with your left arm and left leg, and then with your right arm and right leg.

"I feel beautifully alive in my body and open for energy to flow through my entire being clearly and effortlessly."

ELEVEN *lower body stretches*

Our lower body is involved in most sports and activities (workouts): walking, running, hiking, biking, dancing, skating, and skiing just to name a few. The oscillations in this chapter are perfect to prepare your muscles and joints for these types of workouts, because they increase circulation and range of motion, warming and loosening your body for the workload required. Additionally, all of the oscillations and stretches in this chapter provide a great way to unwind and rebalance your body after your workout.

Lunges

HAMSTRINGS, GLUTES, HIPS, HIP FLEXORS, AND QUADS

WITH TWIST: WAIST, SHOULDERS, HAMSTRINGS, GLUTES, HIPS, HIP FLEXORS, AND QUADS

BENEFITS A well-known stretch to runners, the Lunge provides a deep stretch through a wide range of motion in the hips and legs. By gently pulsing the hip flexor toward the ground you will open the hip flexor quicker than with a still position.

As you twist in the Lunge position, you bring the waist, shoulders, and spine into the stretch. The helps to align the spine and rejuvenate and tone the spinal nerves and ligaments. It also brings more circulation into the abdominal organs and improves the functioning of the digestive system.

• The easiest way to get into the Lunge position is to start on your hands and knees and then bring your right leg forward and extend your left leg back. Align your right knee directly over your heel, and place your hands on the ground next to your foot for support.

• Your weight should be evenly distributed between both legs.

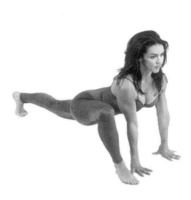

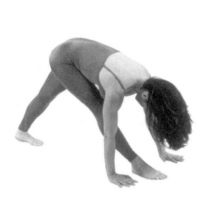

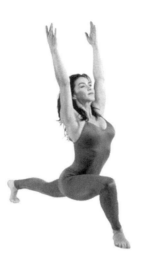

1. Lengthen and straighten your left leg back as much as possible and allow your right hip flexor to sink toward the ground. Gently pulse your right hip flexor toward the ground to increase the stretch.

2. Straighten your right leg with your hands on the ground on each side of your foot.

- Try to keep your hips and shoulders square to the ground.

- Allow your knee to bend slightly if you need to.

3. Reach your arms up to the sky, maintaining relaxed neck and shoulders.

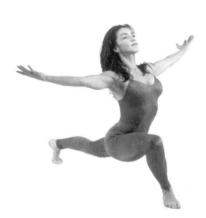

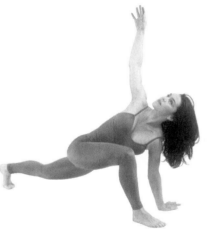

4. Open your arms out to the side, palms to the sky.

Say to yourself: "I am open for all possibilities."

"I am open for all possibilities."

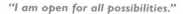

5. Place your left hand on the ground next to your instep.

- Twist to the back, reaching your right arm up to the sky.

- Allow your hip flexor to sink toward the ground.

- Open your heart to the sky.

- Breathe down your spine into your hip.

- Repeat the entire sequence to the other side.

lower body stretches **93**

Knee Lunge

QUADS, HIP FLEXORS, AND GLUTES

BENEFITS This is a great way to get a nice deep stretch for the quads and hip flexors. In this stretch your own body weight assists the depth of the stretch. As you rock side to side the movement increases the flow of energy and fluids into the hip flexor, helping to open the hip joint. Be careful not to go too far. Remember, no further than mild discomfort. With pain there is no gain.

As with any stretch that targets the quads and hip flexors, this is also great for those who run, bike, ski, skate, spin, climb stairs, or do any other activities that involve these muscles. It is also a good stretch for those who sit for long periods of time. I would suggest using this stretch on a softer surface so that your knee is protected. Grass, a rug, or a mat is ideal.

- The easiest way to get into the knee lunge position is to start on your hands and knees and then bring your right leg forward.

SCREAMING KNEE LUNGE

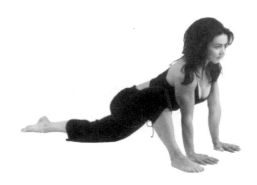
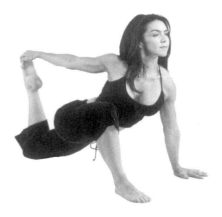

Align your right knee directly over your heel, and place your hands on the ground next to your foot for support.

- Continue to rest your left knee on the ground.

- Let your hip flexor soften as you sink into the position.

- Keep most of your body weight in your front leg.

Draw your left leg in toward your butt.

- Grasp your foot or ankle with your right arm.

- Allow your hip flexor to relax toward the ground.

- Repeat both positions to the other side.

"I walk through life open, aware, and receptive."

Calf Stretch

CALF: GASTROCNEMIUS AND SOLEUS AND ACHILLES, ANKLE, ARCH OF FOOT

BENEFITS Clearing obstructions in the calves opens the way for fresh oxygen and nutrients to circulate through to your ankles and feet. Restoring proper blood flow into these areas becomes increasingly important as we get older. Poor circulation into the feet can eventually manifest into uncomfortable health problems.

I'm not sure who invented heels (probably a man), but for women who wear them they're bad news for the body. And if you're not stretching now, it's definitely time to start. The position that a heel puts your body in is very unnatural; the raising of your heel shortens the Achilles, soleus, and gastrocnemius. This stretch can help you undo what you've done by wearing heels, but be patient. Don't rush through your stretches if you want decent results. Standing in heels for an extended period of time can also put the rest of your body out of alignment. I would highly recommend awarding yourself the time to do a full body stretch to avoid this.

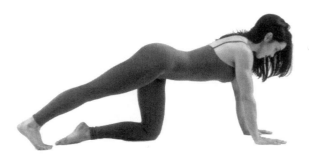 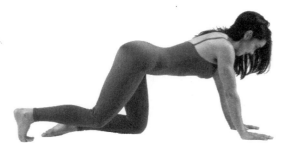

1. Begin on your hands and knees, with your hips directly over your knees and your shoulders directly over your wrists. Extend your right leg back straight, with the ball of your foot firmly on the ground. Press your heel toward the ground, stretching the upper part of your calf, the gastrocnemius.

2. Then bend your leg, continuing to press your heel toward the ground to stretch the lower parts, the Achilles and soleus.

- Repeat these stretches several times on each leg.

"I free myself of attachments and discover blessings of blissful peace."

Pigeon

HIPS, GLUTES, HIP FLEXORS, LOWER BACK, AND INSERTION POINT OF HAMSTRING

BENEFITS Ladies, this is an excellent PMS buster! For those of you who experience symptoms such as lower backaches and cramps—this stretch is a must! Unfortunately our hip flexors, abdominals, and lower back muscles often react strangely to our monthly cycle. By bringing the energy flow to those areas and stretching the muscles that are trying to cramp up, you can combat the uncomfortable feeling in your physical body, which can also help to alleviate some of your PMS blues.

The hip joint is used in just about every physical activity, which places physical stress on the muscles and tendons surrounding the joint. Many people hold emotional stress in these areas, as well. Consequently, tension is often tucked away in the hips and glutes for both men and women. Besides being uncomfortable, tightness in the hips can affect the rest of the body, starting with the lower back and/or knees. This stretch and the Supine Hip Release can prevent and alleviate issues in the hips, lower back, and knees.

- Begin sitting with your legs crossed and then extend your right leg behind you.
- Your right hip flexor, knee, and top of foot should be facing the ground.

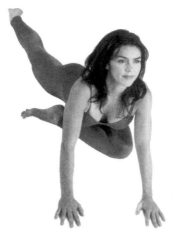

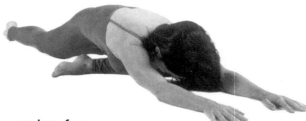

1. Bend your left knee anywhere from five to forty-five degrees (forty-five degrees being the most difficult) and roll toward your left cheek.

- Readjust as you need to in order to feel this stretch in your hip and butt.

2. Lengthen your body forward.

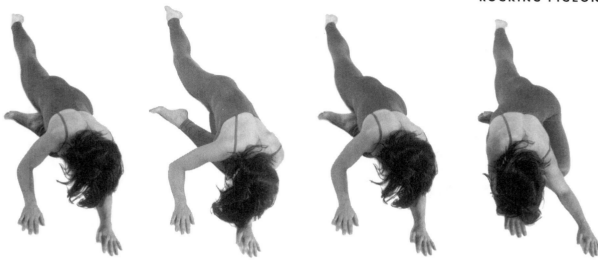

Slowly rock your hips side to side (right and left).

- Move deeper into and out of the stretch each time.

SCREAMING PIGEON

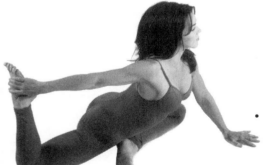

Bend your back leg up, holding your foot or ankle. Gently bring your heel closer to your buttocks. Continue to allow your hip flexor to sink toward the ground.

- Repeat every position you did on the left to the right.

"I am open and willing to let go of anything

blocking or obstructing my flow."

Hip Opener

HIPS, QUADS, HIP FLEXORS, AND HAMSTRINGS

BENEFITS This stretch is nice and easy on the body, and bears great results. This position lying on your side with your knees bent into your chest is usually comfortable for most people.

This stretch opens the hip joint more quickly than most stretches because of the large range of motion it employs. It encourages more energy flow into the target areas, which is achieved at the end point of each position.

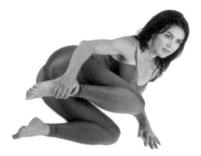

1. Lie on your left side resting on your left forearm with both knees bent into your chest.

- Make sure your hips are stacked directly on top of one another.

- Grab your right foot or ankle.

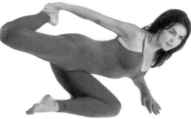

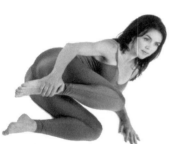

2. Exhale and guide your right leg back, parallel to the ground.

- Stretch it as far as you can comfortably.

3. Inhale as you bring it back to the front.

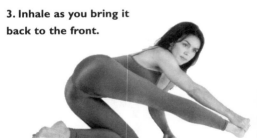

4. Exhale and extend your leg out in front of you.

- Repeat at least four more times (or as many as you'd like).

(This is more advanced. Add it when you feel ready and remember to always work in your own personal range of motion.)

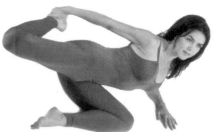

1. Begin with the movement of the Hip Opener and when your top leg is stretched back parallel to the floor you will add the roll.

• Place the inside of your knee on the ground.

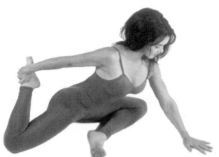

2. Use your hand on the ground in front of you for support.

"I allow my mind and body to experience the bliss of relaxation."

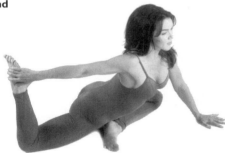

3. Roll your body forward allowing your hip flexor to sink into the ground.

• Gradually roll back in the same fashion and repeat as many times as you'd like to open your entire hip joint (four to eight repetitions usually suffice).

• Repeat every position you did on the right to the left.

Crescent and Half Moon

STOMACH, HIP FLEXORS, QUADS, CHEST, AND SHOULDERS

BENEFITS Both of these positions complement the Forward Bend and the Open Clam. These are not simple stretches, so be easy on yourself when working with these positions. As you move into and out of the position you strengthen your lower back and hamstrings and stretch your abdominals and hip flexors.

CRESCENT

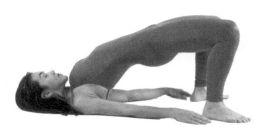

Lie on your back with feet next to your butt. Knees and feet should be shoulder distance apart. Arms should be resting on the ground at your sides. Press your hip flexors up toward the sky.

- Adjust yourself as needed to find your center of balance.
- Take a few BIG belly breaths.

HALF MOON

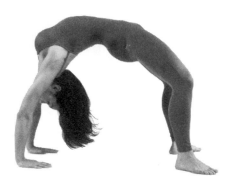

Press up onto your hands if your flexibility allows.

- Optimally (as your flexibility increases) your shoulders are directly over your wrists.

"I keep my heart open to the highest good of all circumstances, as I know

there is a greater plan than my human mind is imagining."

Seated Straddle

INNER THIGHS, HAMSTRINGS, GLUTES, LOWER BACK, WAIST, AND SHOULDERS

BENEFITS The Straddle Circle is one of the most effective ways to go deeper in your straddle stretch. The free-flowing movement of the circle really gets the energy flowing and relaxes the body. Consciously letting go of any gripping or holding on in your body immediately takes down your guard. The legs in particular commonly react to stretches in this position by gripping to protect the body from stretching too far, which blocks the opening of the stretch and can keep you from achieving your optimal flexibility.

This can be considered a more advanced stretch if you're concerned with making a big circle, but the idea is to move gently in your own range of motion, even if it's just an inch in every direction. The smooth movement alone helps the novice or super tight stretcher open in the hips and inner thighs. As with all stretches, work at your own level, don't go beyond the point of mild discomfort, and accept where you are—don't judge yourself.

The roll involves the torso, which helps to flush more energy into the stretch as a whole.

STRADDLE CIRCLE   **Sit in a straddle (legs open as wide as you can comfortably). Circle your body loosely in one direction.**

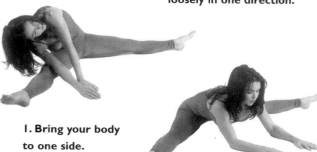

I. Bring your body to one side.

2. Loosely travel through the center.

- Repeat several times on one side and then reverse the circle.

- Throughout the entire circular movement:

  - Let go of any gripping in your thighs and inner thighs.

  - Allow your waist, arms, and neck to be loose and free.

  - Surrender deeper into the stretch with each repetition.

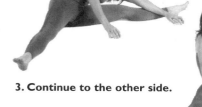

3. Continue to the other side.

4. Then move through the back allowing your torso to contract (round).

STRADDLE ROLL

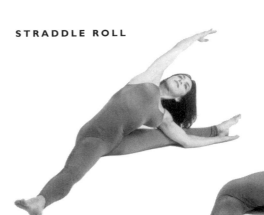

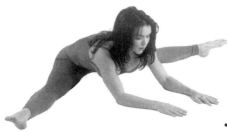

1. Reach your arm over your ear, extending from your hip to your fingertips.

2. Gently roll to the diagonal using your elbows and/or hands on the ground for support.

- Roll as far as you'd like, but not beyond mild discomfort.

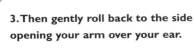

3. Then gently roll back to the side opening your arm over your ear.

- Repeat to the other side.

CENTER REST

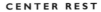

Gently walk your torso forward using your hands on the ground for support.

- Make sure you do not tighten your legs as you take your body forward.

- Consciously release through your hips and inner thighs. Breathe.

"I accept myself exactly where I am right now."

Supine Hamstring

HAMSTRINGS, GLUTES, AND LOWER BACK

BENEFITS This is the easiest and most gentle of all hamstring stretches. With your body weight fully supported by the ground you don't have to concern yourself with balancing or supporting your body. This allows you to focus all of your attention and energy on the stretch. It's very easy to control the amount of pressure put on your hamstrings, since your arms are controlling the stretch.

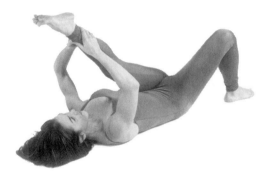

Relaxing on your back: bend your right leg and place your foot flat on the ground.

- Straighten your left leg, bringing it toward your chest.

- Inhale. Release your left leg slightly.

- Exhale. Gently pull your left leg closer to your chest.

- Consciously release your hamstrings.

- Repeat with the right leg.

"I let go of having to be somebody, so

that I can be free."

Supine Hip Release

LOWER BACK, HIPS, AND GLUTES

BENEFITS This is a gentle and comfortable way to stretch the hips and many of my clients' favorite stretch. It's a very easy position to relax in, which always allows for a deeper stretch.

This is also a great hip stretch for those who have knee problems, since there isn't pressure on the knees like you may experience in other hip stretches. Furthermore, many knee problems stem from tightness in the hips, so it is a good idea to keep the hips supple.

The act of softly rocking side to side massages muscles with the movement and feels really good on the lower back and hips. If it is difficult for you to do this in the full Supine Hip Release position, place your bottom foot on the floor for support and indulge in the Rocking Hip Release in a more supported position.

HIP RELEASE

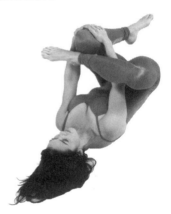

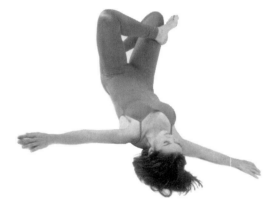

Relax on your back. Cross your right ankle across your left thigh. Bend your left leg and interlace your fingers around your knee. (To modify: hold your left leg behind your hamstring.)

- As you pull your legs closer to your body, flatten your back to the ground.

To modify this position, place your foot on the ground.

- As you breathe allow your lower stomach and lower back to expand.
- Visualize your breath filtering through and cleansing your hip.

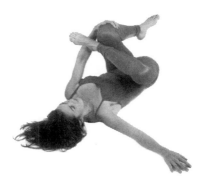

1. Extend your right arm out to the side, palm to the ground for support.

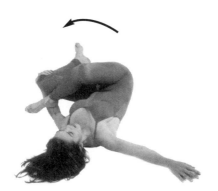

2. Slowly and gently rock your lower torso to one side.

- Allow yourself to go a little bit farther each time.

- Repeat rocking smoothly, side to side as long as your heart desires.

- This is supposed to "hurt so good," but if it hurts in a painful way, try the modified Rocking Hip Release.

- Repeat all positions to the other side.

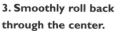

3. Smoothly roll back through the center.

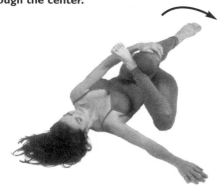

And continue to roll to the other side.

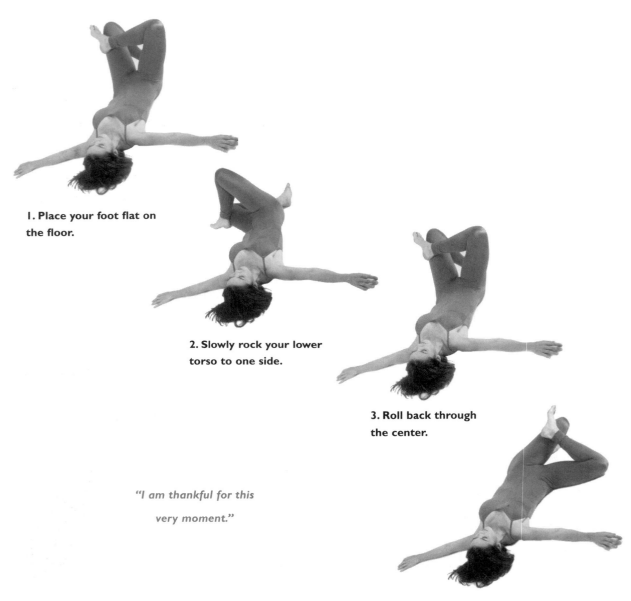

1. Place your foot flat on the floor.

2. Slowly rock your lower torso to one side.

3. Roll back through the center.

"I am thankful for this very moment."

4. Continue the rock to the other side.

- Throughout the entire movement completely relax your hips and glutes.

Lively Feet

CALVES, ANKLES, FEET, AND TOES

BENEFITS Be good to your feet, and don't take them for granted—you rely upon them every day. Keeping them strong, flexible, and agile will help you to enjoy an active lifestyle for many years. These exercises can also improve coordination, movement efficiency, and agility. Circling the foot helps circulation into the lower legs, feet, and toes. This keeps these areas nourished, alive, and well, preventing things like swelling, arthritis, and numbness.

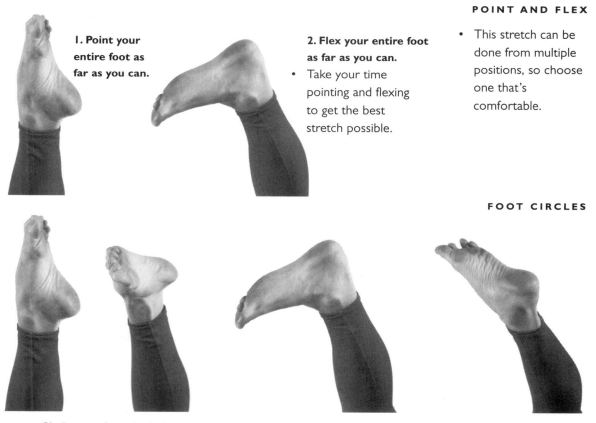

POINT AND FLEX

1. Point your entire foot as far as you can.

2. Flex your entire foot as far as you can.
- Take your time pointing and flexing to get the best stretch possible.

- This stretch can be done from multiple positions, so choose one that's comfortable.

FOOT CIRCLES

Circle your foot clockwise several times. Circle your foot counterclockwise several times.

- Repeat with the other leg, or do both legs together.

"I'm so very grateful for my feet. They have carried me on countless journeys throughout my life."

Child's Pose

BACK AND BUTT

BENEFITS Ahhhh . . . this is a great "chill out" pose. It supports relaxation of the entire body and is conducive to stilling the mind. It is also a great position to visually open the path from the crown to the root. When stress attempts to get the best of you, try relaxing into this pose, breathing deep and calm, allowing your lower back to expand with each breath.

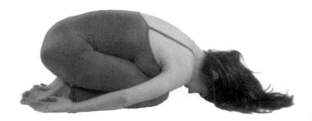

Rest with your knees, shins, and the top of your feet on the floor. Bend forward, relaxing your chest on your thighs and forehead on the ground (you might want to place a pillow under your forehead for added comfort).

- Breathe deeply and calmly allowing your lower back to expand with each breath.

"I simply observe my surface mind-chatter and

let go of the need to entertain it."

TWELVE *upper body stretches*

In this chapter you will find many different upper body stretches that can help you on your road to stress relief and better body alignment. Many people hold mental and emotional tension in the upper body, particularly in the neck and back. Others find themselves with tight muscles from everyday repetitive movements like carrying a purse on one shoulder, lifting heavy objects incorrectly, or sitting stagnantly at the computer. Regardless of where tension comes from, if it's not stretched out it can lead to aggravating kinks, misalignments in the body, and bad posture. To prevent and get rid of tension, consistency is key and a little bit everyday goes a long way. As a reminder, strength training is also important in the quest for good posture and correct body alignment.

Opening Breath

RIB CAGE, WAIST, AND SHOULDERS

BENEFITS One of the most important habits that you will develop through stretching is increasing the power and depth of your breathing. Your breath can effect the way you do everything in your life—not just stretching. Breathing deeply and slowly can be an instant stress reducer, as it calms the nervous system. Any time you feel stress or anxiety coming on, the opening breath is great defense. Most people are shallow breathers. Not only does this make it harder for your body to get the nourishment from the fresh, oxygenated air, but it also feeds anxiety. If you're taking short shallow breaths, you have to breathe more often, causing your body to work harder for less air. If you are accustomed to shallow breathing you may not even realize it, or know that there is a difference, until you become comfortable with calmer, deeper breathing. Do this throughout the day to form a good habit of deeper breathing.

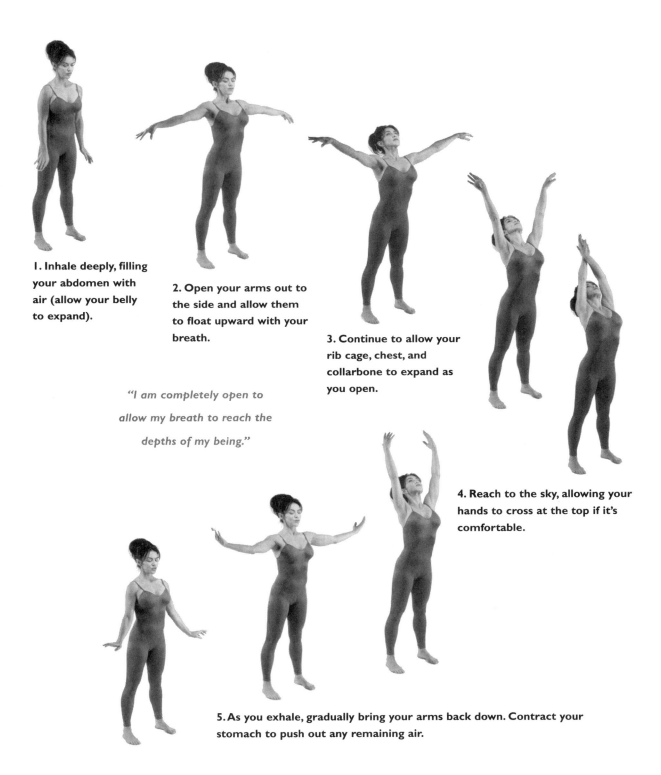

1. Inhale deeply, filling your abdomen with air (allow your belly to expand).

2. Open your arms out to the side and allow them to float upward with your breath.

3. Continue to allow your rib cage, chest, and collarbone to expand as you open.

"I am completely open to allow my breath to reach the depths of my being."

4. Reach to the sky, allowing your hands to cross at the top if it's comfortable.

5. As you exhale, gradually bring your arms back down. Contract your stomach to push out any remaining air.

Half Spinal Roll

NECK, UPPER AND MID BACK

BENEFITS If you tend to carry the weight of the world on your shoulders, this stretch is a must. It stretches and moves energy through the neck and upper back. It's also a great way to get started if you're new to stretching and the Spinal Roll is too much for you. This oscillation can be performed sitting or standing and used for a warm-up before activities, as well as a stress relief stretch throughout the day. Try this coupled with the Half Diagonal Spinal Roll for a quick anxiety buster.

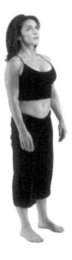

1. Stand straight with your feet shoulder distance apart.

"I meet the day with my heart in the driver's seat."

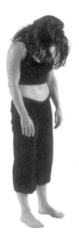

2. Exhale as you bring your chin to your chest.

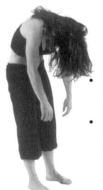

3. Let your shoulders collapse forward.

- Your arms and neck remain loosely relaxed.

- Inhale and roll back up in the same slow fashion.

Half Diagonal Spinal Roll

NECK, UPPER AND MID BACK

BENEFITS This is a simple and quick stretch for those who tend to carry tension and anxiety in the upper back area. It is best when performed after the Half Spinal Roll. The Diagonal Roll reaches farther out from the spine, targeting the trapezius and rhomboids (common housing for anxiety). This stretch is a must for those who work at a computer for long hours.

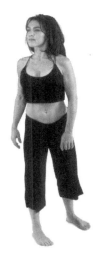

1. Stand straight with your feet shoulder distance apart and turn your shoulders to face the diagonal and inhale.

"I commit myself to keeping my side of the street clean (consciously)."

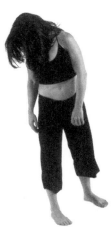

2. Exhale and gently drop your chin to your chest on the diagonal.

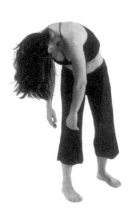

3. Allow your shoulders to collapse as you roll down the diagonal.

- Let your arms and head hang loosely.

- Inhale and roll back up in the same relaxed fashion.

- Repeat to the other side.

Overhead Reach

UPPER TORSO: SHOULDERS, LATS, AND RIB CAGE

BENEFITS Just like a nice breath of fresh air, this is a great anytime, anywhere refresher stretch. It helps to rejuvenate your posture by loosening your shoulders and upper torso. It also restores your breathing by opening your chest and rib cage. This is also a great stretch for your forearms and hands and excellent for those who sit at a desk all day. You don't even have to get out of your seat.

- This can be done sitting or standing.
- Interlace your fingertips.

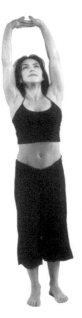

Extend your arms up to the sky.

- Breathe deep and allow your torso to expand with your breath.

"I am grateful for these moments I take to reestablish my clarity."

Shoulder Cross

POSTERIOR DELTS AND RHOMBOIDS

BENEFITS A nice and easy way to stretch your shoulders and part of your upper back without even getting out of your seat. Cross your arm across your body for about ten seconds on each arm to help prevent or relieve stiffness in your shoulders and upper back. Since this takes less than thirty seconds, do it often for greater results!

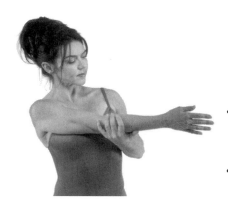

Gently pull one arm across your body at shoulder level.

- Relax your neck and shoulders and breathe into the stretch.
- Repeat on the other side.

"I remember to nurture myself often."

Open Chest

CHEST, ANTERIOR AND MID DELTS

BENEFITS This stretch opens the chest, shoulders, and rib cage and often helps to balance the body. It can improve posture for those of you who have a forward slump. Many people develop a forward slump as they get older due to muscle imbalances and emotional protection. When the shoulders round forward sometimes it is to protect or create an armor over the heart. As you do this exercise, focus into your heart space and allow the energy in your heart to radiate through your chest.

- This can be done standing or kneeling.
- Interlace your finger tips behind your body.
- If you can, keep your palms together.

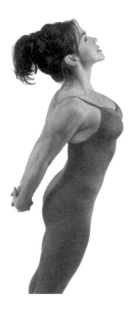

Lift your chest and drop your shoulders.

- Breath deeply allowing your chest and rib cage to expand.
- If you can, raise your arms up in back.

"I open my heart to live from a space of love, not fear."

Overhead Tricep

TRICEPS, SHOULDERS, AND LATS

BENEFITS This is another exercise that can be done while sitting at a desk and does not take much time. This stretch will help maintain elasticity through your shoulders and triceps and keep your reach limber. As we get older, little things like reaching up to get a glass out of a cabinet can become more difficult due to stiffness. Do this stretch throughout the day for best results.

For those of you who lift weights, this stretch is a must. Do this stretch before and after working your triceps.

• This can be done sitting or standing.

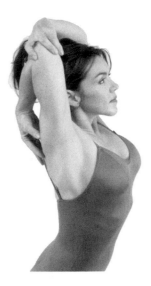

Extend your right arm straight up over your head. Bend your right arm directly behind your triceps. Use your left arm at your elbow for assistance.

• Repeat to the other side.

"I open myself up to greater elasticity and longevity through stretching."

Seated Trap Release

NECK AND UPPER BACK (TRAPEZIUS, REAR DELTS, AND RHOMBOIDS)

BENEFITS If you tend to carry stress in your neck and/or upper back you're not alone. Many people live with "rock gardens," tightly wound muscles, in their tapezius and rhomboids. They can stem from an accumulation of mental or emotional stress such as work deadlines or family pressures, or from an accumulation of physical stress such as lifting and carrying things like babies and groceries. Tightly wound muscles in the upper back can affect the neck, leading to kinks and stiffness and eventually tension headaches. Regular breathing and stretching into these areas can help alleviate tightness and prevent stiffness and tension headaches.

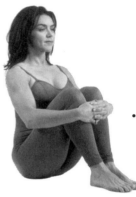

1. Sit comfortably with your knees bent in toward your chest. Interlace your fingertips around your knees.

- You may want to sit on a pillow for tailbone cushioning.

"I allow all my troubles to dissolve back into the illusion where they came from."

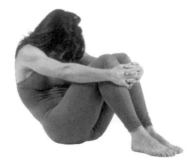

2. As you exhale, round back bringing your chin to your chest. Allow your arms to fully extend to maximize the stretch in your neck and upper back.

- Inhale and come back up into your neutral straight back position.

- Repeat several times weaving your breath into the movement.

Cat Stretch

NECK AND BACK

BENEFITS Stretch like a cat. Get limber like a cat. Tune in to the animal instinct inside of you. Have you ever noticed how often a cat stretches? It's a regular part of their movement and their way of life. Allow yourself to tap into your natural kinesthetic awareness and stretch through life.

The Cat Stretch opens the way for a supple spine, while it strengthens and tones the stomach. It stimulates the ligaments and nerves along the vertebrae, while firing the muscles in the abdominals, trimming the waist.

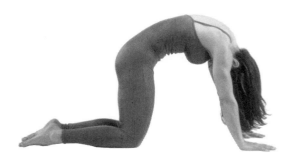

1. Begin on your hands and knees, with your shoulders directly over your wrists and your hips directly over your knees. Contract your stomach in and round up like a cat.

"I open up to my natural kinesthetic awareness and stretch through life."

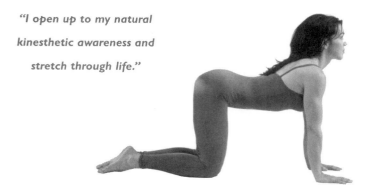

2. Then flatten your back and go into a small arch if it's comfortable.

Lively Hands

WRIST, FOREARM, AND HANDS

BENEFITS Most people don't concern themselves with prevention until it's too late, especially in areas where there is no pain, muscle to gain, or fat to lose. Poor circulation in the forearms, wrists, and hands can lead to arthritis. As we grow older it is increasingly important to keep the circulation flowing into our hands to prevent arthritis. All of these exercises are great ways to get the circulation into the lower arm and hand and increase flexibility. The Fist Burst also increases strength in the hands and forearms.

Additionally these exercises are great for prevention of carpal tunnel syndrome, the "keyboard overuse condition." This condition has put many office workers in casts and braces in the past few years, putting a huge damper on their work and their lifestyle. With society relying more and more upon technology, this condition is becoming extremely common in the workplace. The old-style typewriters required more motion with the arms and fingers, the keys were harder to strike, and the carriage return required movement in the arm. Nowadays, the computer keys are soft and there is no carriage return. One can literally sit in front of the computer and barely move for hours. By taking short breaks to restore circulation to the lower arms, wrists, and hands you can prevent carpal tunnel syndrome. Don't let this epidemic get the best of you—take short stretch breaks periodically while working on the computer.

FIST BURST

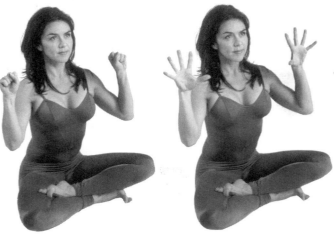

Make a tight fist, then open your hands as wide as possible.

- Do this several times at different speeds.

CIRCLES

- Circle your hands from the wrist clockwise and counterclockwise several times.

"I give my hands the attention they need to stay healthy and lively through my lifetime."

PART FIVE

Essential Stretch
flowing through your life

To say Essential Stretch is an exercise technique is an understatement. To practice Essential Stretch once a week is to miss out on the rich results you can receive by incorporating it into your everyday lifestyle. By taking a moment here and a moment there to focus on your body, you become more alive in your body, yet relaxed and peaceful. By allowing yourself the time to nurture your mind/body/soul connection, you realize your wholeness. By giving yourself just a few minutes a day for breath work and meditation you experience more balance, clarity, and harmony. By weaving Essential Stretch throughout your life, your days become harmonious adventures in love with life.

THIRTEEN *full body routine for getting started*

one Opening Breath

two: Half Spinal Roll

three: Overhead Reach

four: Cat Stretch

five: Calf Stretch

six: Butterfly Contraction

seven: Hip Opener

eight: Clam

nine: Supine Single Leg Hamstring

ten: Child's Pose

One: Opening Breath

The Opening Breath is the warm-up to loosen your lungs and calm your state of being. Breathing is an important part of the stretching process. This exercise prepares you to breathe deeply and calmly while stretching.

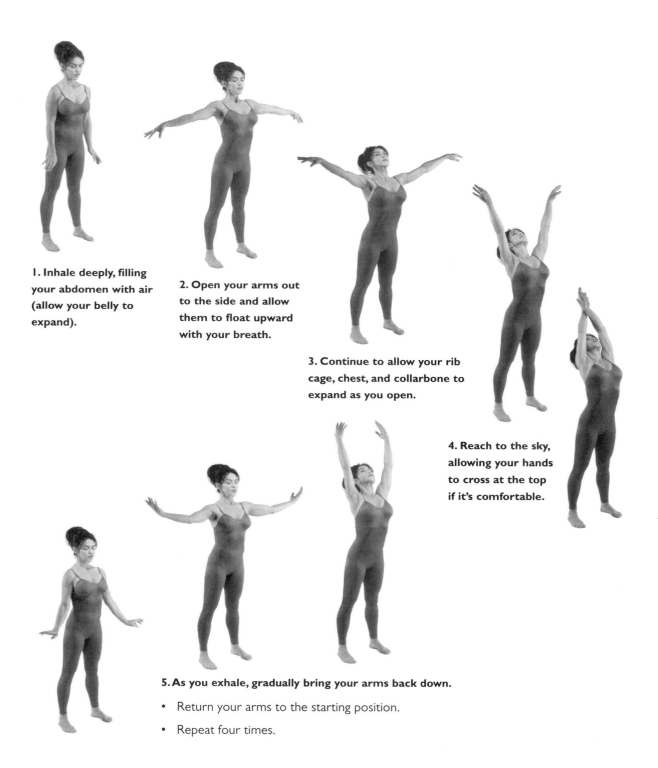

1. Inhale deeply, filling your abdomen with air (allow your belly to expand).

2. Open your arms out to the side and allow them to float upward with your breath.

3. Continue to allow your rib cage, chest, and collarbone to expand as you open.

4. Reach to the sky, allowing your hands to cross at the top if it's comfortable.

5. As you exhale, gradually bring your arms back down.

- Return your arms to the starting position.
- Repeat four times.

Two: Half Spinal Roll *you may do a Full Spinal Roll if it's comfortable for you*

The Half Spinal Roll begins to stimulate the spinal nerves running along the neck all the way down to the mid back. Bring all of your attention to your body and the movement. Breathe down through your neck and spine to encourage cleansing and opening for the free flow of energy. If you choose to do a Full Spinal Roll, continue the focus down your spine to your tailbone.

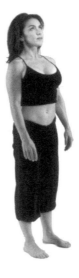

1. Stand straight with your feet shoulder distance apart.

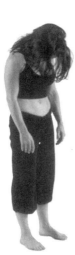

2. Exhale as you bring your chin to your chest.

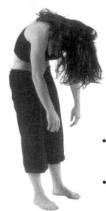

3. Let your shoulders collapse forward.

- Your arms and neck remain loosely relaxed.

- Inhale and roll back up in the same slow fashion.

- Repeat four times.

Three: Overhead Reach

Reach overhead to lengthen your torso and loosen your shoulders. Improving your reach helps you maintain easier movement through daily activities.

- This can be done sitting or standing.
- Interlace your fingertips.

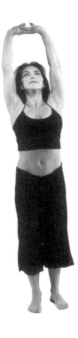

Extend your arms up to the sky. Breathe deep and allow your torso to expand with your breath.

Four: Cat Stretch

Arch up like a cat. Get limber like a cat. Tune in to the animal inside you.

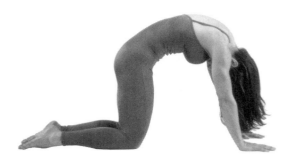

1. Begin on your hands and knees, with your shoulders directly over your wrists and your hips directly over your knees. Contract your stomach in and round up like a cat.

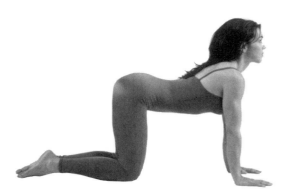

2. Then flatten your back and go into a small arch if it's comfortable.

• Repeat four times.

Five: Calf Stretch

Clearing obstructions in the calf opens the way for fresh oxygen and nutrients to circulate through to your ankles and feet, restoring proper blood flow.

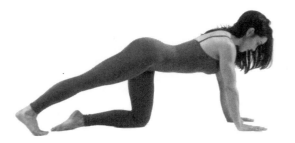

1. Begin on your hands and knees with your hips directly over your knees and your shoulders directly over your wrists. Extend your left leg back straight, with the ball of your foot firmly on the ground. Press your heel toward the ground stretching the upper part of your calf, the gastrocnemius.

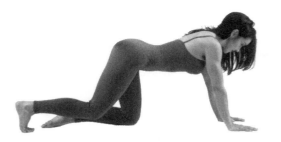

2. Then bend your leg continuing to press your heel toward the ground, stretching the lower parts, the Achilles and soleus.

- Repeat straight and bent on both legs four times.

Six: Butterfly Contraction

The Butterfly Contraction uses the body as leverage to achieve a deeper stretch. Allow yourself to contract back as far as possible, stimulating your neck and spine.

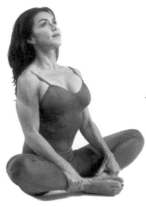

1. Sit tall with your knees open, the soles of your feet together, and your hands grasping your ankles (Butterfly position).

- Lengthen your neck and relax your shoulders down and back.

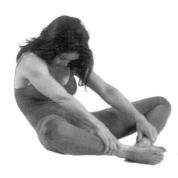

2. Exhale and contract back (rounding your back), bringing your chin to your chest.

- Feel the stretch down through your neck and back.

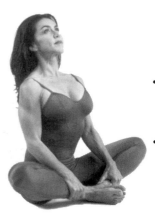

Inhale as you sit back up into your starting position.

- Repeat several times, synchronizing your breath with the movement.
- Repeat eight times.

Seven: Hip Opener

Stretching the quads and hip flexors opens the oxygen flow to the legs. Proper oxygen flow to our legs enables us to walk through life with bounce in our step.

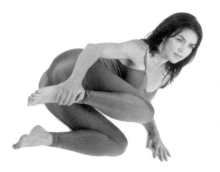

Lie on your left side resting on your left forearm with both knees bent into your chest.

- Make sure your hips are stacked directly on top of one another.

- Grab your right foot or ankle.

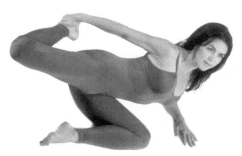

Exhale and guide your right leg back, parallel to the ground.

- Stretch it as far as you can comfortably.

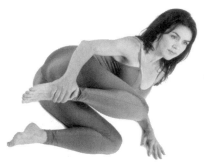

Inhale as you bring it back to the front.

- Repeat four times and switch to the other leg for four repetitions as well.

Eight: Clam

Breathe into each vertebra allowing your back to release tension and stress.

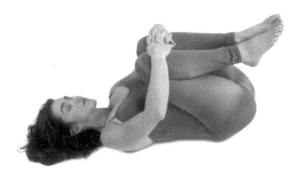

Begin lying on your back and bend your knees into your chest.

- Wrap your hands around your legs.
- Allow your back to melt down into the ground.
- Breathe.

Nine: Supine Single Leg Hamstring

Stretching the hamstrings in this fully supported position permits you to completely relax your muscles. Allow your knee to bend if you need to—you want to feel the stretch in the belly of the hamstring, not behind your knee. If your leg is too far away to grab, use a towel or T-shirt to assist the stretch.

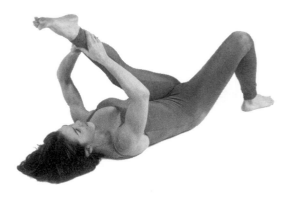

Relaxing on your back, bend your right leg and place your foot flat on the ground. Straighten your left leg, bringing it toward your chest.

- Inhale. Release your left leg slightly.
- Exhale. Gently pull your left leg closer to your chest.
- Consciously release your hamstrings.
- Repeat four times and switch to the other side for four repetitions as well.

Ten: Child's Pose

Finish your stretch workout with a bit of time to be still. This completes your body cleanse as you drop all thought and surrender into the earth.

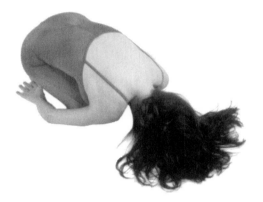

Rest with your knees, shins, and the top of your feet on the floor. Bend forward relaxing your chest on your thighs and forehead on the ground (you might want to place a pillow under your forehead for added comfort).

- Breathe deeply and calmly, allowing your lower back to expand with each breath.

FOURTEEN *full body routine for the seasoned stretcher*

One: Opening Breath

Breathe deeply, opening your rib cage and lungs and allowing your stomach to expand through the movement. This exercise sets you up with the deep breathing that helps your body relax and sink into each stretch.

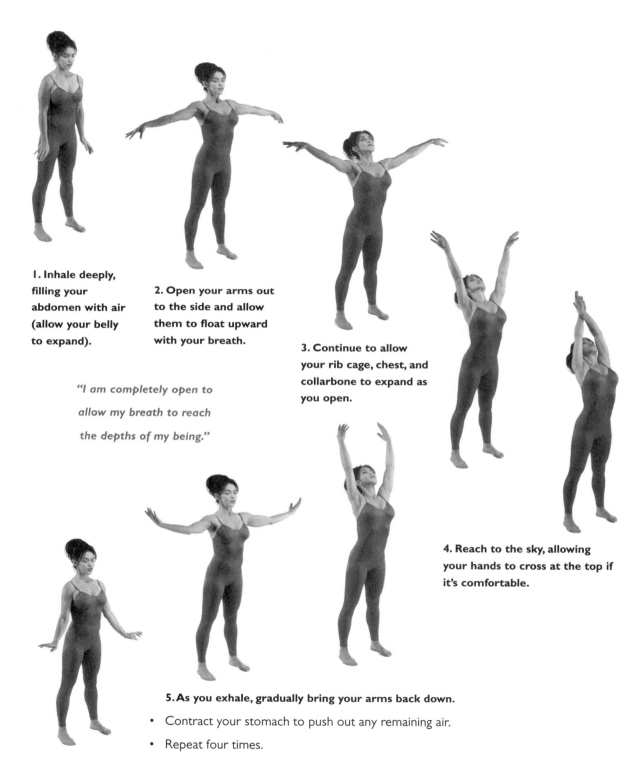

1. Inhale deeply, filling your abdomen with air (allow your belly to expand).

2. Open your arms out to the side and allow them to float upward with your breath.

"I am completely open to allow my breath to reach the depths of my being."

3. Continue to allow your rib cage, chest, and collarbone to expand as you open.

4. Reach to the sky, allowing your hands to cross at the top if it's comfortable.

5. As you exhale, gradually bring your arms back down.

- Contract your stomach to push out any remaining air.
- Repeat four times.

Two: Spinal Roll

Clearing the spine opens the lines of communication to the rest of the body. Breathe down your spine allowing oxygen to replenish the nerves that run down its center. Allow your breath to cleanse blockages and let the energy flow.

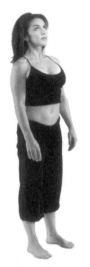

1. Stand straight with your feet shoulder distance apart.

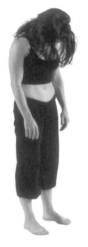

2. Gently bring your chin to your chest.

- Relax the muscles in the back of your neck.

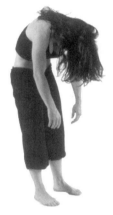

3. Let your shoulders collapse forward.

- Relax the muscles in your upper back, shoulders, and arms.

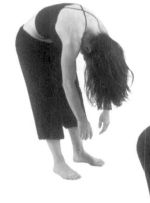

4. Allow your knees to bend gradually as you continue to round forward.

- Relax all the muscles through your back.

- Roll back up in the same slow fashion.

- Repeat four times.

Three: Diagonal Spinal Roll

Allow your arms and head to hang like loose spaghetti noodles (cooked ones!).

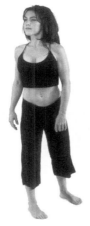

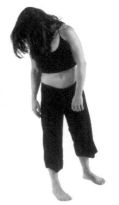

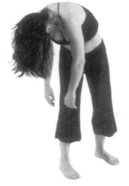

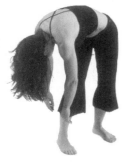

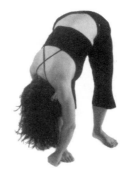

1. Stand straight with your feet shoulder distance apart, and turn your shoulders and hips to face diagonal right.

2. Bring your chin to your chest.

- Let go of the muscles in the back of your neck.

3. Allow your shoulders to collapse forward.

- Let go through your upper back, shoulders, and arms.

4. Continue to roll down through the center of your back.

- Allow your knees to bend and arms to hang loosely, while you relax your entire back.

5. Roll down into your lower back.

- Increase the bend in your knees if you need to.

- Slowly roll up in the same loose fashion.

- Repeat to the left.

- Complete two rolls on each side.

Four: Side Sway

Maintaining a strong center and base, allow your body to freely sway side to side letting your arms and neck be loose and liberal in the movement.

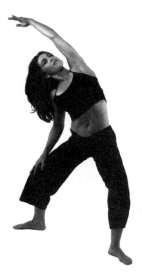

Stand with your legs slightly wider than shoulder distance apart. Feet can be turned out or forward, whatever is comfortable for you. Bend both knees and feel yourself rooted to the ground. Reach your right arm over your head and as far as you can toward the left side.

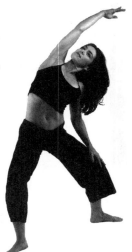

- Use your left hand on your thigh for support.

- Allow your arms to gracefully open as you repeat to the other side.

- Alternate right and left four times.

Five: Multi-level Body Circles

Execute this oscillation slowly for best results. Clearing the clutter from your head to your lower back, this stretch opens you up to much greater mobility throughout your entire torso.

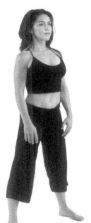

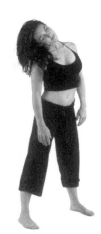

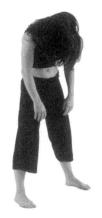

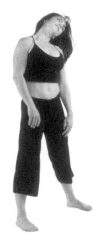

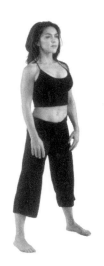

1. Begin by standing with your feet slightly wider than shoulder distance.

2. Gently bring your right ear to your right shoulder.

3. Gradually roll your head to the front.

4. Continue to roll to the left side.

5. And then back to your neutral position.

• Repeat to the other side.

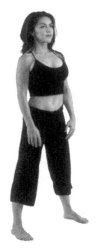

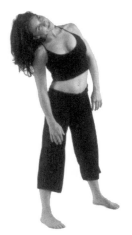

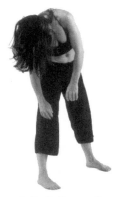

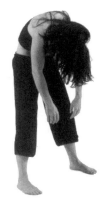

1. Begin by standing with your feet slightly wider than shoulder distance.

2. Gently bring your right ear to your right shoulder.

3. Roll diagonally, allowing your shoulders to collapse forward.

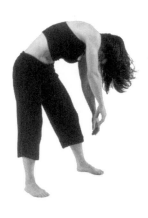

4. Continue to roll through the center and to the other side.

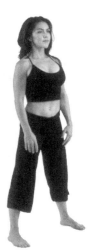

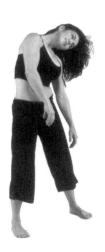

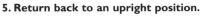

5. Return back to an upright position.

• Repeat to the other side.

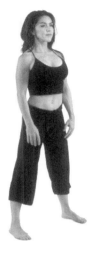

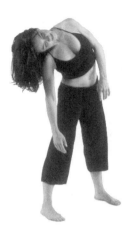

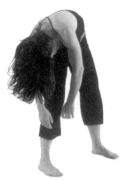

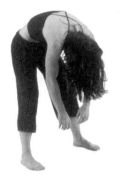

1. **Begin by standing with your feet slightly wider than shoulder distance.**

2. **Bring your right ear to your right shoulder.**

3. **Allow your entire upper back to release to the diagonal.**

4. **Then let go through the center.**

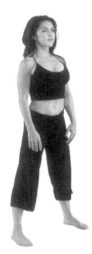

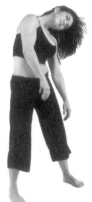

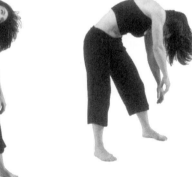

5. **Continue to roll to the other side.**

6. **Return to your upright position.**

• Repeat to the other side.

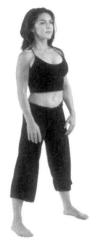

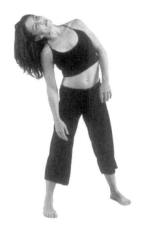

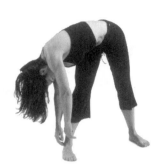

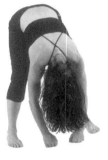

1. Begin by standing with your feet slightly wider than shoulder distance.

2. Bring your right ear to your right shoulder.

3. Allow your entire back to surrender to the diagonal.

4. Smoothly move through the center.

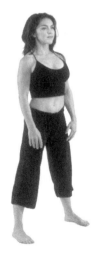

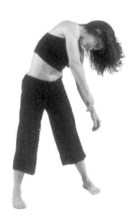

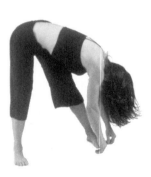

5. Continue to the other side.

6. Rise back up on the diagonal.

7. Finish in your upright position.

• Repeat to the other side.

Six: Lunges

Get the blood circulating throughout your legs, mobilizing your hip joints and clearing the lines of communication into and through your legs.

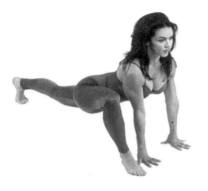

1. Start on your hands and knees and then bring your right leg forward and extend your left leg back. Align your right knee directly over your heel, and place your hands on the ground next to your foot for support. Your weight should be evenly distributed between both legs. Lengthen and straighten your left leg back as much as possible and allow your left hip flexor to sink toward the ground.

- Gently pulse your left hip flexor toward the ground to increase the stretch.

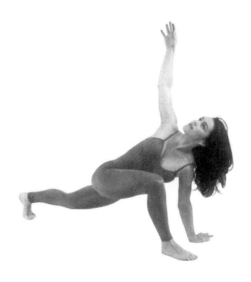

2. Place your left hand on the ground next to your instep. Twist to the back, reaching your right arm up to the sky.

- Allow your hip flexor to sink toward the ground.

- Open your heart to the sky.

- Breathe down your spine into your hip.

- Repeat to the other side.

Seven: Triangle

The Triangle opens each side of the body and some areas of the back. Let go of trying too hard and allow yourself to flow through the movement effortlessly.

1. Begin with your feet in a comfortable wide stance, right foot facing front and left foot facing the side, with your body bent forward at the hips and extended diagonally left. Your left hand is on your ankle or on the ground in front of your foot and your right hand is extended to the diagonal on the ground.

- Allow your head to drop through your shoulders.

- Let go of the muscles in the back of your neck.

- Inhale as you begin to open your body to face front.

2. Inhale as you lift your torso up and exhale as you lengthen your right arm over your ear.

- Lengthen from your hips through your fingertips.

3. Inhale and simultaneously bend your left knee and travel through the center.

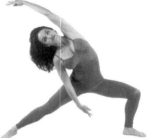

4. Exhale as you reach to the right side.

- Lengthen in your waist as you reach up and over.

5. Inhale as you smoothly open back through the center.

6. Exhale as you straighten your leg and lengthen your right arm over your ear. Inhale as you roll forward towards the diagonal.

- Inhale as you roll forward toward the diagonal.

"I open to reveal the true love, peace, and joy that lies within me."

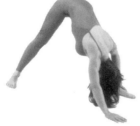

7. Exhale as you relax back into your starting position. Repeat on the other side.

- Repeat three times on each side.

Eight: Rocking Forward Bend

Be free . . . allow your inner child to come out as you roll loosely side to side. This movement opens and nourishes your lower back, hips, and hamstrings.

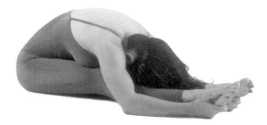

1. Begin sitting with your legs extended straight in front of you and relax your body forward.

- Allow your knees, ankles, and feet to be soft.

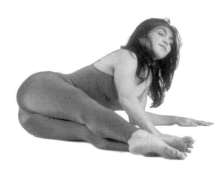

2. Place your hands and elbows on the ground beside your legs for support. Rock your body side to side (left and right). Let your leg and cheek come all the way off the ground.

- Allow your body to sink deeper into the stretch through the movement.

Nine: Seated Trap Release

Smooth out the anxiety kinks. Get rid of the bricks on your shoulders.

- Sit comfortably with your knees bent in toward your chest.
- You may want to sit on a pillow for tailbone cushioning.

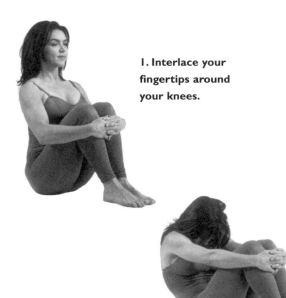

1. Interlace your fingertips around your knees.

2. As you exhale, round back bringing your chin to your chest.

- Allow your arms to fully extend to maximize the stretch in your neck and upper back.
- Keep your shoulders relaxed.

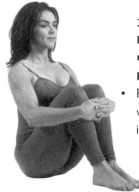

3. Inhale and come back up into your neutral straight back position.

- Repeat eight times, weaving your breath into the movement.

Ten: Butterfly Circle

Close your eyes and allow the movement to take your focus inward.

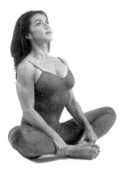

1. Sit tall in Butterfly position.

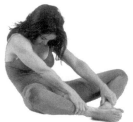

2. Exhale and contract back (rounding your back and chin to your chest).

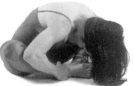

3. Gradually round forward bringing your head toward your feet.

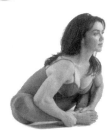

4. Scoop up starting with your head (forehead, nose, then chin), allow your body to follow.

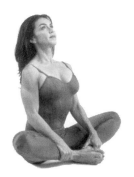

Finish in your starting position.

- Repeat several times.

Eleven: Bird of Paradise

This oscillation lubricates throughout your torso, hips, and shoulders. Feel your body being liberated through the smooth and continuous movement.

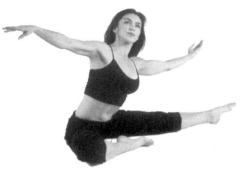

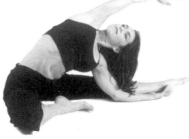

1. Begin sitting with your left leg extended straight out to the side and your right leg bent in. Your hips and shoulders are square to the front. Take a deep breath in and as you exhale, smoothly reach your right arm over your right ear toward your extended leg.

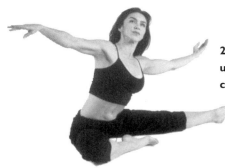

2. Inhale, coming up through the center.

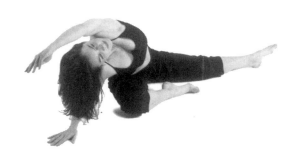

3. Exhale as you reach to the right.

- Continue to weave your breath through the movement, exhaling into the final stretch on each side.

- Repeat to the other side.

ROLL

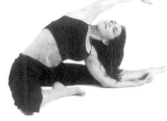

1. Exhale and extend your right arm over your right ear toward your extended leg.

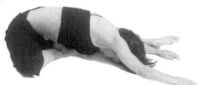

2. Allow your body to slowly roll to the left diagonal.

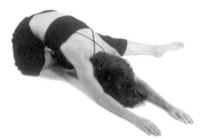

3. Then continue the roll through the center.

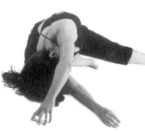

4. And to the right side, to whatever point is comfortable.

• If you can, allow your left shoulder to roll up toward the sky.

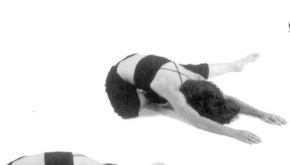

5. Then gradually roll back through the center and to the left and reach your right arm over your right ear.

• Repeat to the opposite side.

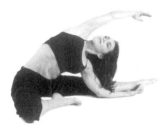

full body routine for the seasoned stretcher **151**

Twelve: Seated Straddle

This oscillation will open your straddle stretch more than ever in a most gentle and comfortable way. The circle raises your energy, while the loose, free movement lubricates the muscles and joints.

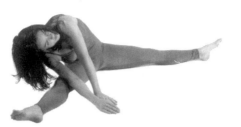

1. Bring your body to one side.

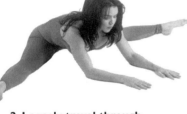

2. Loosely travel through the center.

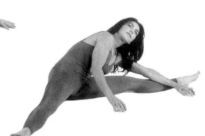

3. Continue to the other side.

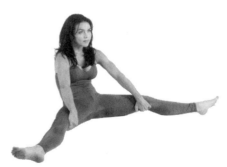

4. Then move through the back allowing your torso to contract (round).

STRADDLE CIRCLE

- Sit in a straddle (legs open as wide as you can comfortably).

- Circle your body loosely in one direction.

- Repeat four to eight times in one direction and then reverse the circle for four to eight circles.

- Throughout the entire circular movement:

  - Let go of any gripping in your thighs and inner thighs.

  - Allow your waist, arms, and neck to be loose and free.

  - Surrender deeper into the stretch with each repetition.

  - Repeat four to eight times in each direction.

STRADDLE ROLL

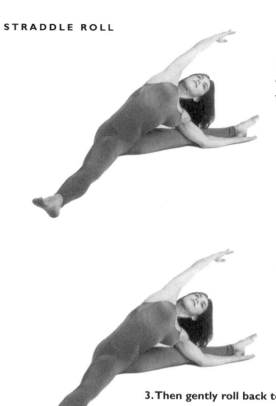

1. Reach your arm over your ear, extending from your hip to your fingertips.

2. Gently roll to the diagonal using your elbows and/or hands on the ground for support.

- Roll as far as you'd like, but not beyond mild discomfort.

3. Then gently roll back to the side opening your arm over your ear.

- Repeat to the other side and do two repetitions on each side.

CENTER REST

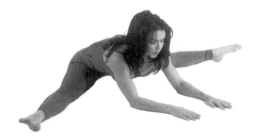

Gently walk your torso forward using your hands on the ground for support.

- Make sure you do not tighten your legs as you take your body forward.

- Consciously release through your hips and inner thighs.

- Breathe.

Thirteen: Rolling Hip Opener

The roll maximizes the stretch in a gentle manner. By incorporating more of the body into the oscillation, energy and fluids are flushed into the hip flexors and quads and open those areas without forcing the stretch.

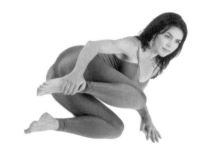

1. Lie on your left side resting on your left forearm with both knees bent into your chest.

- Make sure your hips are stacked directly on top of one another.

- Grab your right foot or ankle.

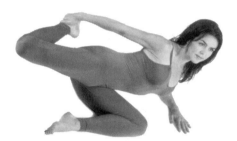

2. Exhale and guide your right leg back, parallel to the ground.

- Stretch it as far as you can comfortably.

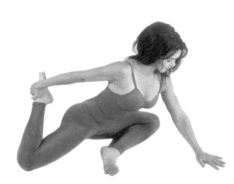

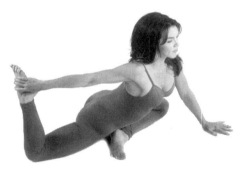

3. Use your hand on the ground in front of you for support.

- Place the inside of your knee on the ground.

4. Roll your body forward allowing your hip flexor to sink into the ground.

- Gradually roll back in the same fashion and repeat as many times as you'd like to open your entire hip joint (four to eight repetitions usually suffice).

- Repeat every position you did on the left to the right.

Fourteen: Supine Hip Release

Free your hips and lower back with this gentle, yet extremely effective oscillation. Allow any troubles you're carrying with you to melt away with the movement.

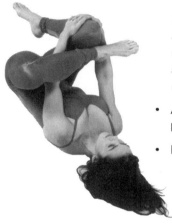

1. Relax on your back. Cross your left ankle across your right thigh. Bend your right leg and interlace your fingers around your knee (to modify: hold your right leg behind your hamstring).

- As you pull your legs closer to your body, flatten your back to the ground.

- Repeat to the other side.

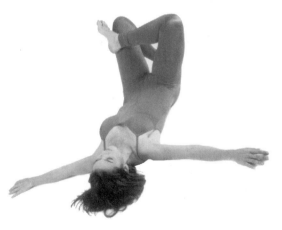

2. To modify this position simply place your foot on the ground.

- As you breathe, allow your lower stomach and lower back to expand.

- Visualize your breath filtering through and cleansing your hip.

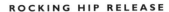

1. Extend your right arm out to the side, palm to the ground for support.

2. Slowly and gently rock your lower torso to one side.

3. Smoothly roll back through the center.

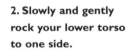

- Allow yourself to go a little bit farther each time.
- Repeat the rock smoothly side to side as long as your heart desires.
- This is supposed to "hurt so good," but if it hurts in a painful way, try the modified Rocking Hip Release.
- Repeat all positions with the opposite leg.

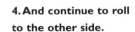

4. And continue to roll to the other side.

Fifteen: Crescent or Half Moon (your choice)

For this exercise, choose between the Crescent and the Half Moon, both of which strengthen the back while lengthening the front. This works the opposing muscle groups as those worked in the Open Clam.

- Lie on your back with feet next to your butt.
- Knees and feet shoulder distance apart.
- Arms rest on the ground at your sides.

CRESCENT

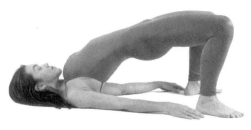

Press your hip flexors up toward the sky.

- Adjust yourself as needed to find your center of balance.
- Take a few BIG belly breaths.

HALF MOON

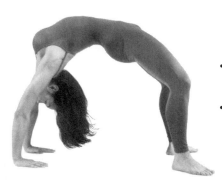

Press up onto your hands if your flexibility allows.

- Optimally (as your flexibility increases) your shoulders are directly over your wrists.
- Alternate the Crescent or Half Moon with the Open Clam two times each.

Sixteen: Open Clam

Smooth out any last little kinks in your back as you use your body for leverage in this stretch.

OPEN CLAM

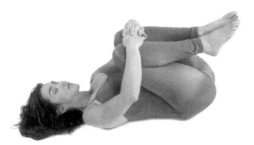

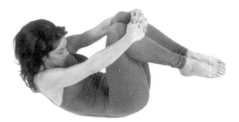

1. Begin lying on your back and bend your knees into your chest. Interlace your fingertips around your knees.

2. Slowly move your knees away from your chest until your arms fully extend. Gradually bring your chin to your chest and raise your upper back off the ground.

- Breathe from your neck down to your tailbone.

- Then slowly flatten your back to the mat.

- Alternate with the Crescent or Half Moon two times each.

CLAM ROLL (OPTIONAL)

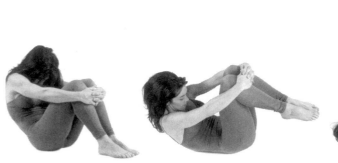

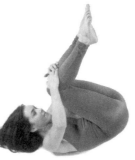

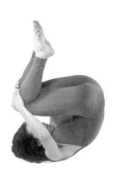

Holding on to your knees, allow your body to roll freely forward and back.

- Smooth and soothe your back through the rock!

Seventeen: Spinal Twist

Rejuvenate the nerves running along the spine. With every breath, simply allow your body to melt into the ground as you follow your breath down your spine.

- Begin lying on your back with both legs extended out straight and bring your left knee into your chest.

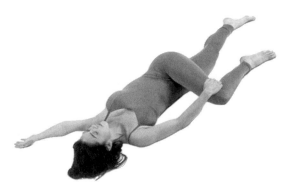

Cross your left leg across your body.

- Extend your left arm straight out to the left.
- Allow your body to melt down into the ground.
- Calmly follow your breath down your spine.
- Rest in this position as long as you would like and repeat to the other side.

FIFTEEN *short and sweet routines*

These shorter routines will help maintain the continuous flow of qi through your body. Inactivity breeds constipation of energy and fluids, which can make you feel stiff and sluggish. Quick stress-relief routines encourage circulation through stagnant areas, mobilize the joints, and stimulate the nerves. These routines are well worth the few minutes you will spend doing them.

Neck and Back Relief

This routine loosens up the neck and back in a very short amount of time. Feel free to do more repetitions of each exercise if you'd like—the amounts shown are designed for you to be able to complete your routine in less than three minutes.

ONE: HALF OR FULL SPINAL ROLL **repeat four times.**

• Open the pathways from your crown to your root.

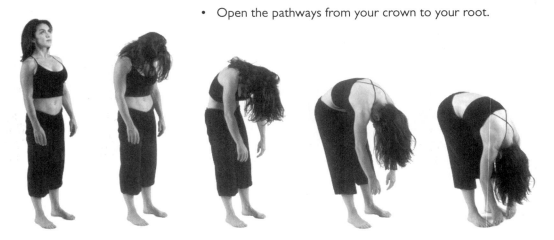

TWO: HALF OR FULL DIAGONAL SPINAL ROLL **alternate twice each side.**

• Allow your breath to be the thread that connects your mind to your body.

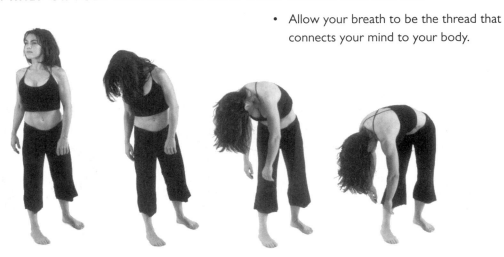

THREE: NECK LOOSENER alternate twice each direction.

- Soothe your neck as you clear the clutter.

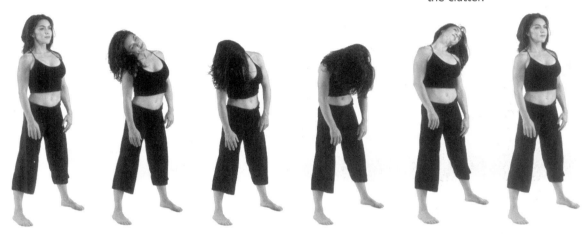

FOUR: UPPER BACK RELEASE alternate twice each direction.

- Roll away the anxiety of the day.

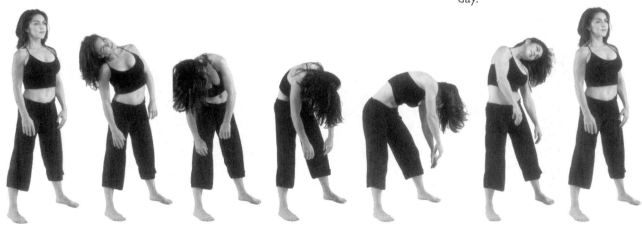

Standing Stress Relief

This one you can do just about anywhere because it doesn't take up much space and you are standing the entire time.

ONE: OVERHEAD REACH/SPINAL ROLL **alternate these two reaching and rolling down and up, repeating four times total.**

- Come alive by clearing the clutter and stimulating the spine.

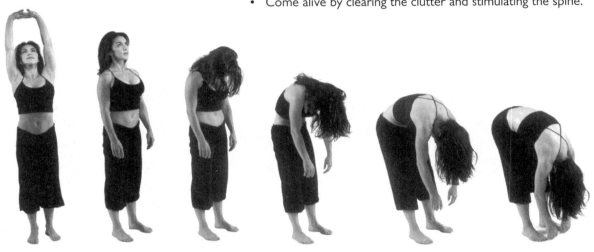

TWO: SIDE SWAY **alternate four times each side.**

- Open your torso, while toning your waist and abdominals.

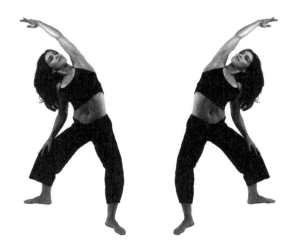

THREE: SINGLE LEG CATERPILLAR repeat four times each leg.

- Strengthen and stretch your back, while lengthening the hamstring and calves.

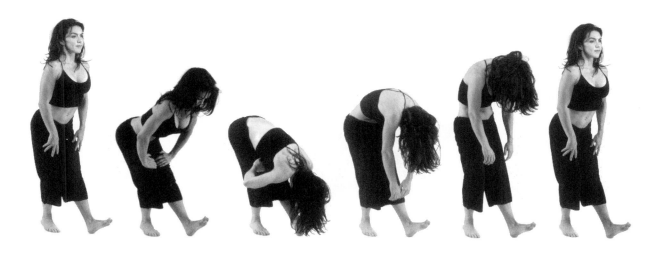

Chill Out

This routine has been developed for those days when you want to loosen up your back and hips, but you're feeling a bit lazy. Listen to your body and give yourself the gift of relaxing back stretches. You may choose to do all of the following stretches, or you may choose to concentrate on just a few. Either way, you're always doing your body some good. So lie down and enjoy!

ONE: CLAM (KNEES TO CHEST) **relax for at least thirty seconds.**

- Set your breathing up during this position, deep and calm.

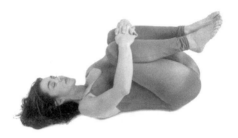

TWO: OPEN CLAM **round up, stretching through your back.**

- Breathe.

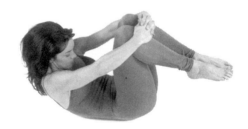

THREE: CRESCENT take three nice, deep belly breaths.

- Allow your belly to fully expand with each breath.

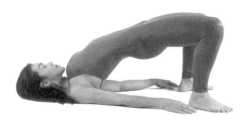

FOUR: SUPINE ROCKING HIP RELEASE repeat both sides for as long as you'd like.

- Massage the muscles with the movement.

Rock left

Rock right

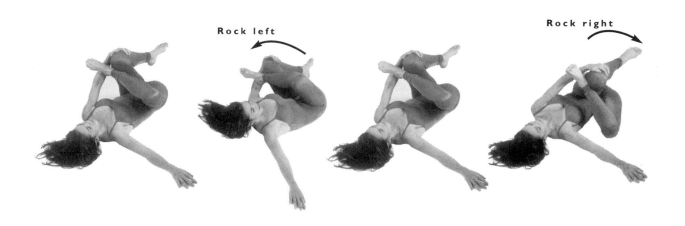

SIXTEEN *daily stretches*

Keep your body feelin' good all day. The following are suggestions to use through your daily journey. Don't limit yourself, get creative—change, rearrange, and add whatever feels right to your body.

Morning Energizers

Honor your body first thing, before you even get out of bed. This will help you start your day from a more open space and a place of peace. After many hours of stillness, Essential Stretches assist in giving your body a gentle wake-up call. This helps your body ease into the day comfortably. Very light stretching is best in the morning.

BODY YAWN (SUPINE EXTENSION)

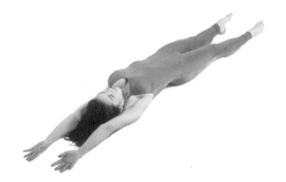

Enliven your body by reaching your arms over your head and extending from your fingertips to your toes. Breathe deep and visualize energy flowing through your body. You can also alternate reaching with your left arm and left leg, and then with your right arm and right leg.

LIVELY HANDS AND FEET

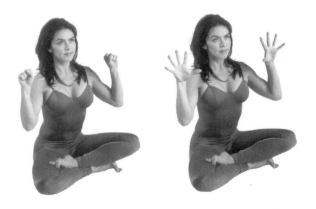

Stimulate your hands and feet by pointing and flexing your toes, and opening and closing your hands.

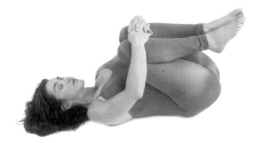

Hug your knees into your chest, gently stretching your lower back. Breathe deeply, allowing your lower back to expand with each breath. If it's comfortable, gently roll side to side. You can do this with your legs opening and closing at each side, or just keep them together the entire time. Do whatever is most comfortable and what feels right for you.

ACTIVATE YOUR HEART THROUGH GRATITUDE

Before you get out of bed, take a moment to focus into your heart space and connect. Rest in gratitude and positive anticipation for the amazing day you have ahead of you. Whatever you need most—creativity, love, joy, wisdom—give thanks for that in advance.

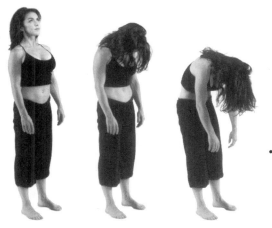

HOT SHOWER STRETCH

1. Take advantage of the warm water beating down on your body and stretch in the shower. Allow the water to warm your neck and upper back as you bring your chin to your chest and round your upper back forward and roll back up.

• Repeat this several times with your neck and back directly under the shower.

Throughout the day fit in as
many stretches as you can.

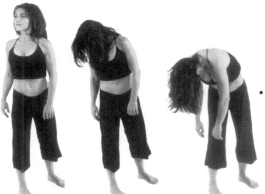

2. Once you feel looser in the center, roll down the diagonal on each side.

• If your body feels loose enough, take these stretches into a Full Spinal Roll and get the circulation flowing through your entire back. It takes some people longer to wake up than others, so listen to your body and do what is comfortable for you.

Desktop De-stress

Sitting for long periods of time can take a toll on your body, especially if your posture is not up to par. Try the following exercise for posture awareness.

POSTURE PERFECT

- Place your hands underneath your bottom where you can feel your sit bones.

- Round back allowing your tailbone to sink down toward the seat.

- Then straighten back up. Notice your sit bones protruding more.

- Notice how straight your back is.

- Relax your neck and shoulders.

- Repeat this a few times solidifying your awareness of how it feels when you have good posture.

Try to maintain that good posture throughout your seated experience. If you feel your posture slump do this exercise again or get up and do some dynamic stretches to revive your body.

Of course, everyone is different and will hold tension in different areas; however, with long periods of sitting most will feel it in the upper and/or lower back.

Upper Back

Stretch as often as you can—every twenty minutes would be great. Do one, two, or all three of the following. These oscillations can be performed seated or standing.

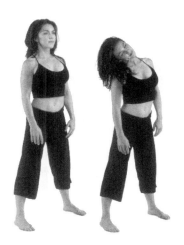 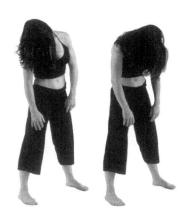 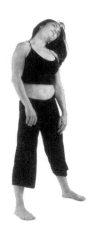 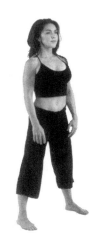

1. Bring your ear to your shoulder.

2. Gradually roll toward the center, taking your chin to your chest.

3. Continue to roll to the other side.

4. Come up to the center (do not roll your head back).

- Repeat to the other side.

- Do not turn your head, your face remains front the entire time.

- Go slowly, allowing tension to melt away through the movement.

- Repeat as many times as you'd like to both sides.

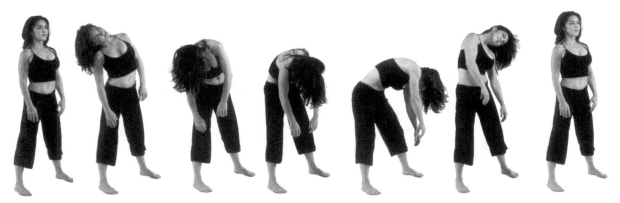

1. Bring your ear to your shoulder.

2. Gradually roll to the center, allowing your shoulders to collapse forward.

- Feel it in your upper back.

3. Continue to roll to the other side.

4. Come up to the center (do not roll your head back).

- Repeat in the opposite direction.

- Again, your face remains front the entire time.

- Focus inward, following the movement with your mind.

- Repeat as many times as you'd like to both sides.

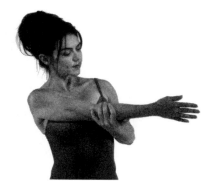

**Bring one arm across
your chest**

- Use the opposite arm to gently pull
  your arm across.

- Feel the stretch in the back of your
  shoulder.

- Repeat to the other side.

Lower Back

Lower back problems are quite common among those who sit for long periods of time. The seated position creates tight hip flexors, which can yank on the lower back. Also, sitting for long periods of time creates stagnation. Getting up out of your seat to stretch periodically is vital. In addition to stretching if you have lower back tightness it is important to strengthen the back and abdominals.

CHILD'S POSE

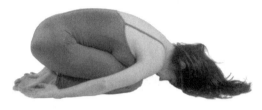

Allow your entire body to relax as you rest on your knees.

- Breathe deeply allowing your lower back to expand with each breath.

HIP OPENER

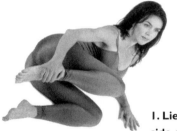

1. Lie on your side and elbow, both knees into your chest.

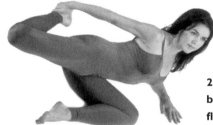

2. Bring your top leg back parallel to the floor.

- Feel the stretch in your quads and hip flexors.

- Repeat this a few times, exhaling into the stretch.

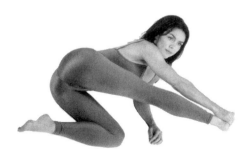

3. As you are ready, add more range of motion (ROM) by bringing your leg forward into a hamstring stretch.

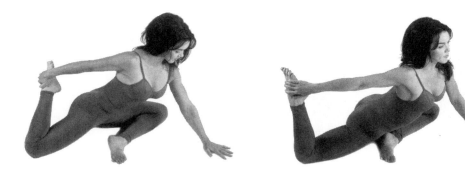

4. To further increase ROM and circulation add a roll forward toward your hip flexor. (This is advanced—do this only when you are ready)

- Repeat this pattern of movement as many times as you need.

Forearms, Wrists, and Hands

LIVELY HANDS

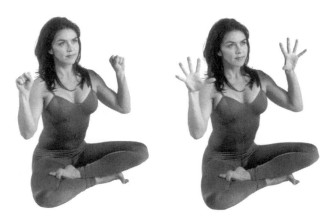

If you're tickling the keyboard for more than thirty minutes, your hands will adore a good stretch. And though you may not think you need it, carpal tunnel syndrome is making its way to dominating workplace physical therapy practices. So it's wise to take preventative measures. Every so often take your hands off the keyboard and make a fist then open it, fist, open, fist, open—several times. If you have time, get up and walk around while you're doing this.

Mother's Refresher

Moms—have you ever felt like your well has run dry? With all your attention focused on family matters—laundry, changing diapers, shopping, cooking—when is your time to replenish? Sometimes all you need is some time to nurture your soul, to be by yourself without being pulled in ten million different directions.

While the baby's asleep, instead of jumping into chores that need to be done, take the first five minutes (or more) for you. Choose your favorite stretch and perform it with a deep inward focus, like a movement meditation. Let your heart smile in gratitude for this time you've given yourself. Though you may not feel like you have the time, it will replenish your well and provide you with blessings you may need.

"Stretching makes my mind clearer, more able to handle chaos. I used to get nervous that I wouldn't remember everything 'cause I have so much to do, but when I take the time to stretch I come from a more relaxed space and I seem to remember everything really easily."—ANNETTE, MOTHER OF THREE, IN NEW JERSEY

Traffic Anxiety Busters

DEEP BREATHING

- Breathe in through your nose as deep as is comfortable.
- Allow your stomach to expand with your breath.
- Hold that breath in for just a few seconds.
- Exhale slowly.
- Try to make your exhale last longer than your inhale.
- Repeat as often as needed.

STOPLIGHT STRETCH

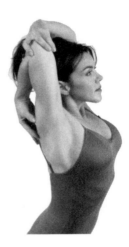

Extend your elbow up to the sky.

- Use your opposite hand to gently stretch your lat and tricep.
- Breathe into the stretch and don't forget to do both sides.

Jet Lag Reducer

Prevent the travel kinks while energizing yourself for your trip. Stretch before, during, and after your flight. This will help you be more comfortable in your seat and arrive more refreshed. It's optimal to do a full body stretch either before or after a long flight; however, since time and location may not always permit such a luxury, a little stretch is better than none.

While you're flying:

LOWER LEGS, ANKLES, AND FEET

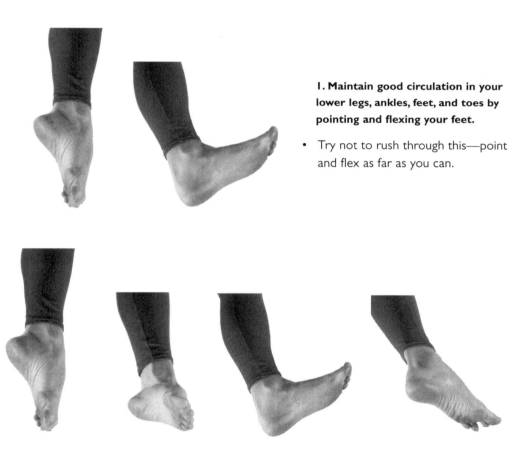

1. Maintain good circulation in your lower legs, ankles, feet, and toes by pointing and flexing your feet.

• Try not to rush through this—point and flex as far as you can.

2. Then circle your feet clockwise and counterclockwise.

• Again, take your time.

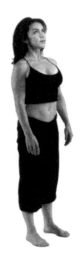
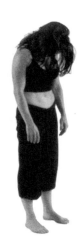

1. Exhale as you bring your chin to your chest.

• Allow your shoulders to collapse forward.

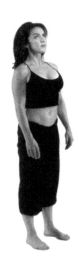

2. Then inhale as you roll back up to a straight position.

• You can also do neck and upper back circles in your seat. (See Desktop De-stress.)

OVERHEAD REACH

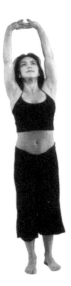

Interlace your fingertips and lengthen your arms.

And for those of you who want to stretch more while flying, go to the back of the plane and stretch (as long as the seatbelt sign is not illuminated and the flight attendants don't object). Stretches such as the Side Sway, Spinal Roll, and Diagonal Spinal Roll are good ones for small quarters. See Chapter 10 for detailed explanations.

Bedtime Relaxers

Stretching before you go to bed at night will not only help you get a more restful sleep, but can also makes a big difference in your mental and physical clarity the next day. The best stretches to do at night are different for each individual. You want to target those areas where you hold the most tension. For everyone, the Spinal Roll is a great start, and this may be enough. But for those of you who want to feel even better, get down on the floor and go for it. Bring your breathing into a deep and calm state, slowing your system down for a peaceful sleep. If you're doing oscillations, do them very slowly. If you're doing still poses, allow your body to sink deeper with each breath.

Choose your favorite bedtime stretches from Part Four. Here are some of my favorites.

STANDING CATERPILLAR—(DETAILED INSTRUCTIONS PAGE 70)

BUTTERFLY CIRCLE—(DETAILED INSTRUCTIONS PAGE 84)

BIRD OF PARADISE—(DETAILED INSTRUCTIONS PAGE 81)

SEVENTEEN *mind your mind*

put your awareness into action

As you increase your sensitivity through stretching, you become more keenly aware of where you hold tension in your body. This body knowledge comes gradually through the process of stretching. To facilitate the process, while you are stretching take note of those areas that feel tight. When you encounter a stressful situation, observe your body. Do you feel any particular part of your body tensing up? Do you feel stiff or tight later on that day or the next and where? By observing your body through life's trials and tribulations you are gathering knowledge to counter the effects of stress on your body.

Increased mind/body awareness also helps us discover those things that ignite tension in our body. We call these our stressors. Sometimes stressors come from exterior sources and sometimes they come from the inside—our ego's creations. External stressors are things like a crabby boss, screaming children, or even preparing for a party at your house—not all stressors come from what you might consider negative circumstances. Internal stressors can come from insecurity about your physical appearance or abilities, worry about the future, or carrying around baggage from the past. No matter where it's coming from, the key is recognition. As you become more aware you will be more cognizant of the stressors that set off a charge in your system. Shallower breathing; a tense feeling in your neck, back, or entire body; nervous twitching; inability to clear your mind; sternness in your face; and clammy hands and feet are all signs of stress entering your system. Sometimes signs are subtle and other times they're obvious, but the more in tune you become, the easier it is to identify your stress monsters. This gives you power to sidestep the effects of stress by taking action right away.

on the spot active relaxation

As a reminder, it is most important to create a peaceful internal atmosphere with daily stretching and meditation, but stretching is also a great way to combat stress. When you feel stress coming on, consciously breathe deep and slow and do your favorite oscillation to stretch the area where you are holding stress. For years wellness experts have been promoting the use of belly breathing for overall health and stress reduction. "Deep breathing from your diaphragm causes a natural relaxation response, lowering your heart rate and blood pressure," says Timothy Moore, a health and fitness consultant from Santa Monica, California. "Short of doing some type of physical activity, it's one of the best ways to help relieve the effects of stress on your body."

If you're in a situation where you can't break out into a full stretch, continue to breathe deep and if possible excuse yourself and retreat to a place where you can. If you're on the phone and the voice on the other end has got your blood boiling ask if you can call them back, then center yourself with a few concentrated oscillations. By taking care of yourself when necessary and not waiting until later, you can help to counter the affects of stress on your body. How many times have you said to yourself, "I'll relax later" or "I'll meditate later" and then it never happens? Just a couple minutes can provide a positive change in perspective and that may be just what you need to get back in your flow.

insecurity zapper

We all have our moments. So when you're feeling blue or not good about yourself, give yourself a huge loving hug. Then, with your arms wrapped around at the level of your heart, close your eyes and focus into your heart. Take nice, slow, deep breaths into your heart space, allowing your rib cage to expand with each nourishing breath. Do this for at least sixty seconds. You may notice some thoughts swimming across your mind. As this happens, bring those thoughts into your heart and just be.

This can be done standing, sitting, or lying down. Do this as many times as you would like. The more you do it, the easier it gets to tap into your heart and truly hear the wisdom it has to share.

stop the insanity

When negative thoughts are swimming rapidly through your mind, with worry, doubt, or fear taking over—stop and stretch! This is your chance to overcome or rise above fear-based mind-chatter. Each time you connect your mind to your body, you shift your focus and create the opportunity for a shift in consciousness. The mind and body work together and completely affect one another in positive or negative ways. If you do something repetitive and your body develops a kink from that repetition, your mind oftentimes will respond with frustration. Likewise, if your mind is attacking you about some issue, whether it is insecurity, worry, doubt, or fear, it will eventually manifest in the body. The mind and body are not separate. They feel the negative effects of stress together, just as they feel the positive effects of stretching together. So when you recognize your mind's imagination going wild, try not to entertain those thoughts. Instead, get out of your head by doing your favorite oscillation. Focus on your body intently.

Then if you'd like, focus on your heart. When you feel sufficiently connected, ask for your fear-based consciousness to be dissolved through the stretch.

step up concentration (between tasks or anytime)

Ever find it hard to concentrate when you have to switch gears all the time? Say you're putting together a proposal and you take a phone call, putting your attention on something completely different. Then maybe a colleague comes by your desk and puts something else in your mind and so on until you've completely lost your focus on the proposal. Just as you would cleanse your palate between courses, cleanse your mind between projects and distractions with a quick stretch. This will bring closure to what you were doing and help you center so you can go back to your project or prepare for the next thing on which you must focus. For optimal results, treat these movements like a movement meditation, very slowly with a strong focus inward.

Dear Reader,

I bless you on your Essential Stretch journey and hope that you continually discover the richness of self-awareness and openness to life. This is not necessarily an easy journey, especially in the beginning, but a very rewarding one. I can say for myself that Essential Stretch has completely changed my life and continues to help me grow on my spiritual journey. When I look back to where I was when I began my quest to heal my body, I realize I was like a type-A, stressed out, chaotic Energizer Bunny. After more than ten years of peeling back many layers of physical, mental, and emotional stress through Essential Stretch, I feel peaceful, grounded, and very awake and aware with beautifully focused energy. Having more calm, focused energy has helped me in all aspects of my life, from easily creating hot choreography to communicating more clearly with others. Each of you will be rewarded in your own unique way and I wish you the very best on your journey.

    Namaste,

    Michelle

notes

Chapter Two

1. Corliss, Richard. "The Power of Yoga." *Time*, April 23, 2001, pp. 61.
2. Wilson, Stanley D., Ph.D. *Qi Gong for Beginners*. (Portland, OR: Rudra Press, 1997), 6.
3. ——————, pp. 5.
4. ——————, pp. 6.
5. Aerobics and Fitness Association of America and Reebok. *Fitness Theory and Practice*. (Sherman Oaks, CA, and Stoughton, MA: University Press, 1997), 325.
6. Andes, Karen, with the editors of *Fitness* magazine. *Fitness Stretching: Mind, Body, Spirit*. (New York: Three Rivers Press, 2000), 16.
7. Goldberg, Ken, M.D. "Help for Erectile Dysfunction." WebMD Corp., 2001.
8. The National Institute of Diabetes and Digestive Kidney Diseases of the National Insti-

tute of Health. "All About Impotence." Publication no. 95–3923, March 16, 1998. http://niddk.nih.gov.

9. Yoga International Reprint Series. *Simply Relaxing.* (Honesdale, PA: Himalayan Institute, 1998), 6.

Chapter Three

1. Bauman, Brint, and Piper Wright. *The Holistic Health Handbook.* (Berkeley, CA: Berkeley Holistic Health Center, 1978), 372.

2. Wayne, D. "Reactions to Stress." In Identifying Stress: A Series Offered by the Health-Net and Stress Management website, February 1998. http://healthnet.com.

3. Childre, Doc, and Howard Martin. *The HeartMath Solution.* (New York: HarperCollins Publishers, 1999), 57.

4. Weinart, Jerry, and Jill Bielwaski. *Stretching for Health.* (Chicago, IL: Contemporary Books, 2000), 40.

5. *Fitness Stretching*, 18.

Chapter Six

1. Corliss, Richard. "The Power of Yoga."

2. Yoga International Reprint Series. *Yoga.* (Honesdale, PA: Himalayan Institute, 1994), 2.

Chapter Seven

1. Childre, Doc, and Howard Martin. *The HeartMath Solution*, 6.

2. Armour, J., and J. Ardell, eds. *Neurocardiology.* (New York: Oxford University Press, 1984).

3. Childre, Doc, and Howard Martin. *The HeartMath Solution*, 69.

index

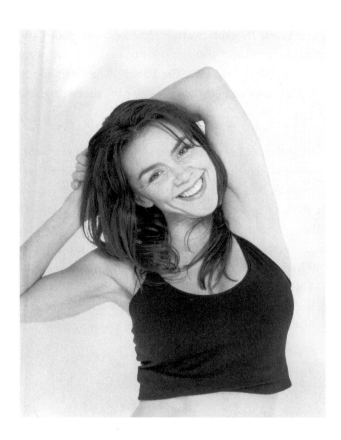

about the author

Michelle LeMay is a world-renowned fitness expert and dance choreographer who develops movement techniques designed to enhance personal growth, self expression, and peak performance in life. Known as the "instructors' instructor," she has shared her methods with thousands of fitness professionals via her series of interactive workshops. Michelle has spread her inspirational training techniques throughout the United States, Canada, Mexico, Japan, Brazil, Argentina, Spain, Singapore, Malaysia, Indonesia, Germany, Luxembourg, Russia, Italy, Belgium, Switzerland, and Greece.

Michelle has also shared her training methods with millions through TV shows and videos. She was costar and choreographer for ESPN II's *Gotta Sweat*, and FOX Sports/FITTV's *Body Waves*. Michelle has hosted a number of dance workout videos and has also cohosted several video series with six-time Ms. Olympia Cory Everson and actress/workout guru Jane Fonda. Michelle is instantly recognizable to television audiences from her many appearances as a fitness expert on ABC, CBS, USA Network, and The Family Channel, among other media outlets. Additionally, she was a health and lifestyle reporter for more than five years for the CBS affiliate in Tampa.

LeMay is known for her innovative teaching techniques and unique approach to movement, which incorporates the whole person—mind, body, and soul—resulting in deeper and longer-lasting results than traditional fitness training. Many of her students call her classes "movement therapy," as she has taught them to release their stress and the burdens of life while nurturing mind, body, and soul through movement. LeMay believes dance, exercise, and stretch can be extremely healing and emotionally uplifting with the right approach and the right attitude. Through her past affiliations as a spokesperson for companies such as RYKA, NIKE, American Fitness, and Mademoiselle, she has inspired millions of people to step out of their box, experience new techniques, and grow to their next level. Whether she is training one-on-one or teaching a class of thousands, LeMay has the uncanny ability to draw out the best in people.